50 Things that Cause Earache

Dr Yagyadut Gupta

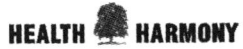

An imprint of
B. Jain Publishers (P) Ltd.
USA — EUROPE — INDIA

50 THINGS THAT CAUSE EARACHE

First Edition: 2012
1st Impression: 2012

All rights reserved. No part of this book may be reproduced, stored in a retrieval system or transmitted, in any form or by any means, mechanical, photocopying, recording or otherwise, without any prior written permission of the publisher.

© with the author

Published by Kuldeep Jain for

HEALTH HARMONY

An imprint of
B. JAIN PUBLISHERS (P) LTD.
1921/10, Chuna Mandi, Paharganj, New Delhi 110 055 (INDIA)
Tel.: +91-11-4567 1000 • *Fax:* +91-11-4567 1010
Email: info@bjain.com • *Website:* **www.bjain.com**

Printed in India by
J.J. Offset Printers

ISBN: 978-81-319-1139-6

Dedicated to

My Late Father, Shri Sant Lal Gupta...
My constant source of inspiration

Publisher's Note

The book – *50 things that cause earache* – is written in a straightforward and lucid manner, enriching one's knowledge from the basic to the intricate ear problems – faced by the society, today. In trying to move on with life we often lose our sense of direction regarding 'what all' to keep in mind to make life simpler and free of troubles.

Today people young and old comprise such major chunk of population who carry on with the new electronics as an inseparable part of their lifestyle. The latest i-pods, earphones, bluetooth – all these basically prove hazardous to the human ear. Dr Yagyadut Gupta tries to bring to us an awakening of the reader about all the harmful as well as fatal aspects regarding ear problems. The book oozes with all types of relative information regarding the human ear and its problems. It serves as a gift from the author to the society.

Kuldeep Jain
C.E.O., B. Jain Publishers (P) Ltd.

Foreword

Science is exciting, but medical science is even more exciting as it deals with the study of the human beings.

The present day world is growing with new technological advancements. So, it is quite natural for anyone to get mislead, particularly for the ones who do not have the complete awareness of the medical field.

So, it is very important for the people to have proper knowledge and information regarding how to go about getting right treatment in case of ear problems.

After going through the book I found that 50 Things that Cause Earache – is a humble and sincere effort in the direction to provide all types of information regarding ear problems – in its basic, easy and lucid form. The book is very appropriate and important guide for all ear patients.

I congratulate the eminent and promising Otorhinolaryngologist, Dr Yagyadut Gupta, for making this information available for the people of the society. For a non-medical person this is going to be an interesting reading material.

Dr Harish Gupta
MD (Medicine)
Consultant & Associate Professor
Department of Medicine,
PGIMER & Dr Ram Manohar Lohia Hospital,
New Delhi
Physician VVIP Medical Unit,
Prime Minister Office/House

Preface

'No work is done without hard labour.'

– Swami Vivekananda

Earache, though seems to be a small thing, is ultimately a very difficult thing to get diagnosed. I have put in my years of effort on ear point patients so as to make them overcome their problems. Their trust in my work has made me author this book today. So, it really feels pleasure to recall and quote – Swami Vivekananda – who always stressed upon 'work' and its importance in the success of a human life.

The graph of the patients with ear problems is growing day by day, with the advent of new technological advancements. The growing excitement in the youth of today to make the new electronics an important part of their lifestyle – has proved to be very dangerous. The growing use of cell phones; i-pods; blue tooth devices; ear phones – are not only the cause of ear problems but they basically lead to – loss of hearing. So, definitely electronic should be used in a limited way so as to enjoy a happy life.

The intense air travels in the city civilization, today, are also a major cause of a lot of ear problems, later on leading to sinusitis and throat problems.

This book is a major guide, educating ear patients with various treatment modalities and simplifying things for future quick recoveries.

The major target of this book is to point out the predominant reasons of the causes of an earache, and how fatal its negligence can be!

Dr Yagyadut Gupta

Acknowledgements

First of all, I thank my Almighty God who has bestowed his love and affection on me throughout my life and has given me the best. It is by His grace that I am writing this book and will try to make few things easier for common man to understand about the various ear problems.

This book is dedicated to my late father, Mr Sant Lal Gupta, who had been a constant source of inspiration for me. He was a perfectionist and always believed in simple living and high thinking. His ideology, hard work, helping attitude, honesty and smiling face is the force behind my working also.

My mother, Mrs Taramani Gupta, is also a constant thinker for the betterment of my life. She has an untiring attitude and always yearns for my success. Without her power, persuasion and firm belief in God, I would not have come so far. She has worked behind the curtain for my achievements in life.

Dr Sshally Gupta, my better half, has given me the strength to overcome the obstacles in my growth and has inspired me to succeed in my profession. Her silence says everything and she, again, constantly works for my success.

My daughter, Yashii and son, Aadityaa, give me the best time of their lives and a reason to smile when I come back from work. Their smiling faces make me more energetic and provide me with a new zest to work.

I wish to thank my family members, friends, relatives and well wishers for praying for my success in my profession.

I am trying to reach to the common man and make things simple for them regarding the various problems of earache encountered by them in their day to day life. I hope I will succeed in my attempt to ease out few matter related to ear diseases.

At last, I will feel satisfied when my book is appreciated by the readers.

Dr Yagyadut Gupta

Contents

Publisher's Note   iv
Foreword   v
Preface   vii
Acknowledgements   ix

Chapters

1. Introduction   1
2. Anatomy and Physiology of the Ear   7
3. 50 Causes of Earache   11
4. Dos and Don'ts when you have an earache   153
5. Simple Tips to Take Care of Your Ears   159

Chapter 1
Introduction

50 Things which can Cause Earache

Pain in any part of the body, especially, in the ears is

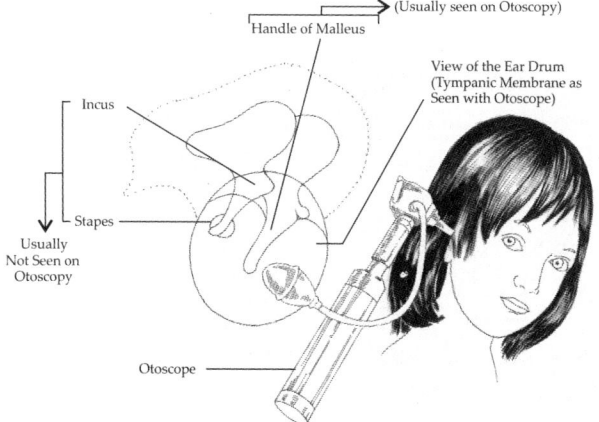

Fig. 1.1 Examination of the Ear Canal (External Auditory Meatus) Using Otoscope

very troublesome. It causes a lot of distress to the person along with loss of working hours. It is very important that being a physician one understands the distress the other person is going through, in pain. The physician's feel, of the amount of the immense pain, the patient is undergoing, makes the curing much more easier. The doctor examines and clears the disease of the patient, keeping in mind that if he himself had to undergo the same procedure in pain, how much stress could he have undergone.

Ear pain comparatively is very stressful. It happens due to many reasons such as – infection in the ear, or it may be precipitated because of an infection in the nose, throat, dental or any other region. People apply various ways to get rid of the pain but when they are not successful only then they come to see a doctor. The general tendency seen is – the use oil, use of urine of different animals, use of various ear drops and juice of onion – to get relief.

People have a tendency, rather they have deep rooted old beliefs that a particular method of treatment will be effective for all kinds of pain in the ear. One such method is instillation of warm or hot oil in the affected ear. It is difficult to make them understand that one method which may be helpful for a particular type of disease may not be applicable to all types of problems in the ear. In spite of repeated warning to patients; putting up articles in newspapers and using other methods of awareness among them still it is difficult to change their mindsets.

Ear pain is at times easy to treat if we find the root cause of it or at times it becomes difficult if that cause is not picked up. Nevertheless, once the proper diagnosis is done its treatment becomes simpler. Pain in the ear can make a child cry throughout the night and can leave the parents restless through the night. At times parents do not understand that the child, who is not able to speak, is crying because of pain in the ears. They think there may be other reasons for the pain and come late for an ENT inspection.

The pain in the ears may not be directly linked to the ear pathology only and it may be referred from adjoining structures like scalp, neck, nose, teeth, parotid gland, temporomandibular joint and larynx. Then it is called REFERRED pain. We are collectively citing the 50 causes of ear pain in this book i.e. directly linked because of ear pathology and referred pain from the adjoining tissues.

These many things and the varied presentation and severity of ear pain inspired authoring this book for the common man. This book can create a general awareness of the various conditions in and outside ear which can cause ear pain and it would be handy for them to understand and treat the condition accordingly by themselves or by proper consultation. This is not a medical jargon but a book in simple language for the benefit of common man.

50 things or causes which produce ear pain are as under.

Causes of Ear Ache (Otalgia)

1. Impacted Wax
2. Furunculosis or Otitis Externa
3. Acute Otitis Media
4. Perichondritis
5. Mastoiditis
6. Otomycosis
7. Herpes Zoster Oticus (Ramsay Hunts Yndrome)
8. Facial Nerve Palsy Trauma
9. Trauma to the Ear
10. Acute Tonsillitis
11. Dental Caries
12. Submandibular Lymphadenitis
13. Barometric Trauma during Scuba Diving and Seafloor Walking
14. Mumps
15. Apthous Ulceration

16. Ludwig's Angina
17. Malignant Otitis Externa
18. Foreign Bodies in the Ear
19. Dermatitis of the External Ear
20. Haematoma of the auricle
21. Osteoma of the External Auditory Canal
22. Aural Polyps (Ear Canal Polyps)
23. Cholesteatoma
24. Acute Sinusitis
25. Carcinoma of the Ear (Pinna)
26. Cerebellopontine Angle Tumour (Acoustic Neuroma)
27. Quinsy
28. Retropharyngeal Abscess
29. Acute Cervical Lymphadenitis
30. Diptheria
31. Iatrogenic
32. Otosclerosis
33. Glomus Tumours
34. Carcinoma of the External Auditory Canal and Middle Ear
35. Elongated Styloid Process (Eagles Syndrome)
36. Glossopharyngeal Neuralgia

37. Infection in the Preauricular Sinus
38. Torticollis
39. Temporo-mandibular Joint Syndrome
40. Cancer of Larynx
41. Goitre
42. Cervical Spondylosis
43. Vocal Cord Nodules (Teacher's or Screamer's nodules)
44. Whiplash Injury to Neck
45. Artificial Dentures
46. Pain in the Ear during an Aeroplane Flight
47. Use of Earphones
48. Herpes Simplex of the Oral Cavity
49. Leucoplakia of the Oral Cavity
50. GERD
51. Migraine

Before going ahead, it is important to understand the anatomy of the ear canal and its adjoining structures. The following chapter explains this with nice illustrations. Understanding the anatomy of the ear is a bit difficult but we have kept it simpler for the common man to understand.

Chapter 2

Anatomy and Physiology of the Ear

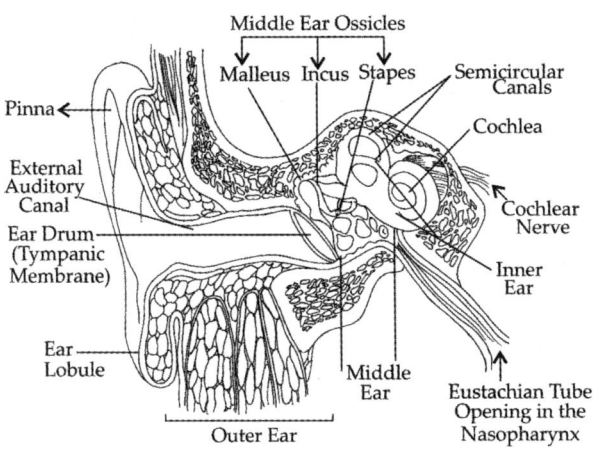

Fig. 2.1 Cut Section of Right Ear External Auditory Canal

Anatomically, the ear can be divided into three parts:

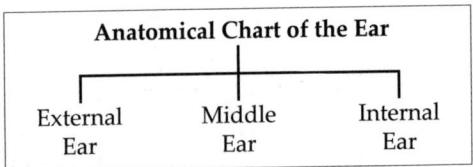

Fig. 2.2 Anatomy of the Ear

1. **The external ear** It consists of the pinna and the external acoustic meatus. The external acoustic meatus is about 24 mm in length and has hair and ceruminous glands in its outer third region. Outer third region is cartilaginous. Inner 2/3rd is bony and is devoid of hair and ceruminous glands.

   Note: The furuncles in the outer third of the cartilaginous acoustic meatus are extremely painful due to increased tension in the tissue.

2. **The middle ear** It is the part of the temporal bone. It is a six-sided box with anterior-posterior, medial-lateral and superior-inferior walls.

   Anteriorly, the Eustachian tube connects it with the nasopharynx. Posteriorly, it is connected with the mastoid antrum. The facial nerve in its horizontal course lies close to the posterior wall.

   Medially cochlea (promontory) lies along with the round and oval window. Oval window is closed by the foot plate of stapes.

Anatomy and Physiology of the Ear | 9

Laterally, the middle ear is closed by the tympanic membrane or tympanic membrane forms the lateral boundary of the middle ear.

Superiorly, the roof of the middle ear is the tegmen tympani which separates the middle ear from the middle fossa of the skull.

Inferiorly, the floor of the middle ear is separated from the internal jugular bulb by a thin plate of bone.

The most important part of the middle ear are the three bones – malleus, incus and stapes – which are the integral part of the hearing system and help in the conduction of sound waves from the external to internal ear. The other content is air.

Stapes is the smallest bone in the body of human beings which lies over the oval window. Middle ear helps in the equalisation of the air pressure during the pressure changes as are seen during the takeoff or landing of the flights.

Note: Infections from the nasopharynx travels to the middle ear via Eustachian tube opening. Mastoiditis or the infection in the mastoid part of temporal bone happens because of infections in the middle ear. The facial nerve is at times damaged in the surgery of mastoid in cases of unsafe chronic suppurative otitis media. It is in the promontory, that the hole is done and cochlear implant part is pushed in the cochlear implant surgery in hearing impaired patients. Tympanic

> membrane may be ruptured due to infections in the middle ear leading to acute or chronic suppurative otitis media conditions. Duramater (lying in the roof of the middle ear) may be damaged during mastoid surgery especially when it is low lying, by which iatrogenic infections may pass from middle ear to the brain. High jugular bulb may be exposed and may be damaged during the middle ear surgeries. The ossicular chain being the integral part of the hearing system may be damaged leading to loss of hearing due to infections of the middle ear.

3. **The internal ear** It lies in the petrous part of the temporal bone. It comprises of cochlea and three semicircular canals (lateral, posterior and superior).

   The three semi-circular canals are connected to the vestibular component of the VIII cranial nerve (i.e. vestibule-cochlear nerve) and the cochlea is connected via the cochlear component of the VIII cranial nerve.

   The vestibular and cochlear components of the VIII cranial nerve help in the balancing of the body and hearing, respectively.

> **Note:** The fistula in the lateral semi-circular canal due to unsafe Chronic suppurative otitis media leads to disturbance in the balance of the body and may lead to development of the vertigo (spinning of the head). Its in the promontory (overlying Cochlea), a hole is done and hearing aid part is pushed in cochlea in the cochlear implant surgery in hearing impaired patients.

Chapter 3

50 Causes of Earache

The chapter explains the 50 causes of Earache. The discussion of each cause of the earache accompanies its reasons; symptoms; the necessary treatment and its prevention.

Impacted Wax

Generally, the wax formation occurs in the ear due to the ceruminous glands or sebaceous glands. Ears have got small hairs whose rhythmic movement pushes the wax out of the ear. Thus the self-cleaning mechanism of ear keeps the ear clean.

Reasons: Using of ear buds pushes the wax inside the ear and results in impaction of the wax. Wax may also get accumulated due to faulty self-cleaning mechanism. The advert use of oil and use of car keys – increases the risk of infection and impaction of wax.

Presentation (Signs and Symptoms): Patients normally come with sensation of blocked ears, heaviness in the ears, hearing loss and at times pain. The onset is often sudden following swimming, bathing or washing when the water entry in otherwise narrowed ear canal closes the ear by swelling of the wax. At times, it is just found at the time of ENT examination without any symptoms. Pain in the ear usually happens due to – use of hot oil, ear buds infection following swimming in the pool, river or sea.

Treatment: Ear cleaning under direct vision is the best way to remove the impacted wax. Other methods of ear cleaning like syringing with warm water or by use of vacuum suction may also help in cleaning the loose wax.

Prevention: Never use ear buds at home to clean the ear, it will further push the wax inside and lead to impaction and pain in the ear. Use of warm oil (Olive oil, Almond oil or Mustard oil) may be used with caution under confirmed presence of wax in the ear. It helps in softening the wax in these patients. This may relieve the pain temporarily if the wax is too much impacted. Warm or hot oil use in otherwise not too healthy and the already clean ear may result in perforation of the ear drum or infection. Use of urine of animals or self at times, as has been seen in my practice, should be absolutely contraindicated.

Furunculosis or Otitis Externa

(Infection in the external ear): Outer third of the external ear canal has hairs. It is in these hairs that infection can get embedded and may lead to severe pain.

Reasons: Normally during bathing, swimming, river rafting and scuba diving, water goes inside the ear canal and comes out. Normally it dries up and does not lead to infection. But in hot and humid conditions particularly, moisture may sit in the ear canal hairs and lead to infection. This may cause severe pain due to the tight attachment of the ear skin in this region. At times, impacted wax with the movement of water inside the ear canal may set in the infection and lead to furunculosis or otitis externa.

Presentation (Signs and Symptoms): These patients usually present with severe pain in the ear which is more so on chewing food, eating and/ or opening of mouth. Children may present themselves with fever or with crying day and night without any obvious reason in the other parts of the body. Mothers may often say that the child starts crying the moment they touch or pull the ear/s. Even feeding on the affected side is not comfortable with the child and so may not take feed on the affected side.

There is no obvious pus seen on examination of the external ear in most of the cases. Usually, there is narrowing of the ear canal in comparison to the normal size of ear and there is severe pain on pulling the affected ear upwards and outwards for examination. Patients should be handled very gently in this condition. Slight bending of the pinna or external ear may also produce excruciating pain. Apart from pain, there is usually no pus discharge seen. In few of the patients, pus may be seen in later stages.

Treatment: Wax should be cleaned gently under vision in cases with impacted wax condition. Ear cleaning of the wax with the syringing method using warm water may be avoided in this condition. Usually, Icthymol Glycerol ear pack with the gauze piece improves the condition. This pack may need to change every second or third day for at least two to three times for complete resolution of the infection. Proper oral antibiotic coverage along with strong analgesics may be required along with the ear pack for early resolution of the disease. Pack need to be prevented from getting wet during the treatment period. Chances of re-infection are high in rainy and humid conditions particularly during monsoons.

Prevention: Frequent use of ear buds for cleaning should be avoided. Hot fomentation of the affected ear further aggravates the problem and should be contraindicated. Swimming, river rafting and scuba diving may cause the condition in a few. Improper use of ear drops without consultation should not be done. In children, where there is no obvious cause of crying, this condition should always be ruled out by showing to the ENT consultant.

Acute Otitis Media

Acute Otitis Media is the infection of the middle ear. Middle ear is the part of the ear which forms a partition between the external ear and the internal ear. Middle ear is connected to the nose and throat via Eustachian tube. Infections from nose and throat contribute to most of the infections of the middle ear. Middle ear contains the ossicles which helps in transmission of the sound and helps in the hearing process. Infections of the middle ear damage the ossicular chain and leads to the hearing loss also. Middle ear is separated from the external ear via tympanic membrane, rupture of which may result in infection reaching to the middle ear.

Reasons: Infection in the middle ear happens due to infection travelling from nose and throat region. Tonsils, adenoids, sinus infection are the main culprits for acute otitis media. Barotrauma caused by scuba diving, sea floor walking or diving in the swimming pool may also be responsible for this condition. Travelling by air also causes pressure changes in the ear and especially during descent with associated cough and cold may lead to increased pressure in the ear leading to acute otitis media. In newborns and infants faulty feeding habits (breast feed, top feed) in head low position may cause the feed to move into the eustachian tube and subsequent infection of the middle ear. Foreign bodies in the ear like insects, mosquitoes, ball bearing balls and peas – may induce infection in the external and middle ear as well.

Presentation (Signs and Symptoms): Patients of acute otitis media present themselves with the complaint of pain, heaviness, decreased hearing, and popping sensation in the ear, at times unsteadiness, giddiness and ear discharge. These symptoms may be present according to the severity of the disease.

Congested tympanic membrane (Reddish ear drum) with or without bulging of the ear drum is usually seen in this condition. Pus may be seen bulging in severe acute otitis media on otoscopy. Patients usually have running nose with white or yellowish discharge as seen in common cold or sinusitis.

Treatment: Conservative management is commonly required in management of the acute otitis media. Broad spectrum antibiotics, anti-allergics, pain killers and cough suppressant are the usual medicines to be taken according to the need of the patients. Ear cleaning may be required if ear discharge is present and swab may be sent for culture and antibiotic sensitivity. Instillation of the ear drops required if ear discharge is present. Uncommonly, ear drum is surgically incised (Myringotomy) and fluid or pus drained out with putting ventilation tube in the ear drum (Grommet Insertion). New ear drum may be surgically repaired if the ear perforation persists (Tympanoplasty).

Prevention: Prevention is better than cure. The old dictum stays true in these cases, also. Proper management of cough and cold, i.e. acute adenotonsillitis, acute tonsillitis, acute sinusitis, acute pharyngitis, influenza helps in prevention of acute otitis media in most of the cases. Mothers should be trained for appropriate breast and top feeding practices. Traumatic perforations should be handled aggressively and avoidance of oil and ear drops instillation helps in curing most of these cases. Scuba diving, swimming, diving, sea floor walking, and air journey should be done with caution in patients suffering from cough and cold.

Perichondritis

'Chondr' in medical terminology stands for the cartilage. Infection of the cartilaginous part of the ear, i.e. pinna is called as Perichondritis. Cartilage has the property that once its get infected it loses its shape unlike bone which maintains its shape if properly treated in time. So the cartilaginous infection of the ear is often associated with the deforming of the ear. Cartilage injuries and infection are difficult to treat and these are annoying to the patient and treating physician since the results are mostly unsatisfactory. These most of the times cause cosmetic deformity of the pinna which is difficult to correct.

Reasons: Perichondritis is commonly seen in boxers, wrestlers and road-side injuries. It may be seen as a complication of ear piercing or as a result of boil/abscess in the external ear canal spreading to the pinna. Injury to the ear (Pinna) causes collection of the blood between skin and cartilage which results in impairment of the blood supply to the cartilage resulting in its deformation.

Presentation (Signs and Symptoms): Patient usually present themselves with severe pain and tenderness on palpation. The ear pinna becomes stiff on touching and is not that freely mobile as in normal condition. Perichondritis is often seen with swelling on both sides of the ear with loss of shape of the pinna. Blood collection on the surface of the ear produces bogginess which is compressible and soft on touch. The temperature of the swelled ear is raised on palpation.

Treatment: Initial treatment consists of broad spectrum Antibiotics, Analgesics. In few of the cases, Incision and Drainage of the swelling and compressible bandage with antibiotic ointment impregnated gauze filled in the cavity is done. Even with best of the treatment, necrosis of the ear cartilage may cause loss of normal contour of the ear. At times, post treatment haematoma gets solidified and becomes permanently embedded in the soft tissues, giving a permanent cauliflower appearance of the pinna as is seen in boxers and wrestlers.

Prevention: Wearing helmets while playing boxing or wrestling prevents the development of perichondritis. Using helmets while driving bike, scooter or cycles prevent the same from happening. Proper management of outer ear boil or furuncle should be done at the earliest so to prevent the development of perichondritis.

Mastoiditis

Mastoid is the region behind the pinna. Its close association with the middle ear is important since the infection from the middle ear can spread to the mastoid, especially, in children and in repeated ear discharge cases in adults. Mastoid is underdeveloped in the newborns and facial nerve lies more open in its vertical course. Chances of facial nerve damage on surgery are more in children due to the absence of developed mastoid.

Reasons: Mastoiditis happens due to the spread of infection from the middle ear to the mastoid. The pus travels from the middle ear cavity to the mastoid process in the absence of adequate treatment. Acute otitis media is the main condition which leads to the infection of mastoid with subsequent development of mastoiditis. Mastoiditis may happen rarely due to the penetrating injuries to the mastoid or road side accidents. Mastoid is a tough bone and infection is difficult to reach from outside sources in normal circumstances.

Presentation (Signs and Symptoms): Infection in the mastoid usually presents with pain and swelling behind the ear. Affected ear is displaced anteriorly and outward. Pus may travel in different directions:

- If it travels down it may travel towards the upper neck.
- Anteriorly it may travel towards eye causing eyelid swelling
- It may travel upwards causing intracranial (Brain) complications.
- It may move toward the ear canal and present as discharging furunculosis.

There is usual presentation of ear discharge, loss of hearing and fever. Pain on palpating the region of mastoid is a common finding.

Treatment: Conservative management with broad spectrum antibiotics has already decreased the incidence of mastoiditis. But still it is common in suburbs and low hygienic areas. Acute mastoiditis with pus and mastoid swelling not resolving with the antibiotics is dealt surgically. An incision is given behind the ear in the region of mastoid and pus is drained out. Care is taken not to put the incision too anteriorly near the ear so to prevent damage to the facial nerve especially in the children. Proper opening up of the mastoid process is done in adults and cortical mastoidectomy is performed in them.

Prevention: Prevention of mastoiditis depends upon the awareness in the community regarding the development of acute otitis media which in turn depends upon the morbidity of cough and cold in the society. So actual prevention is of cough and cold which eventually leads to mastoiditis. Ear discharge may not be present in all cases of mastoiditis (Masked Mastoiditis) so even if the fever and hearing discomfort with pain in the mastoid region is present then even adequate consultation with an expert is necessary.

Otomycosis

'Oto' stands for the ear and 'mycosis' stands for the fungus. Thus fungal infection of the ear is called otomycosis. Fungal infection is common in the ear as in the other parts of the body.

Reasons: Fungal infection in the ear is seen in hot and humid climate. People involved in activities like swimming, sea walking, scuba diving, water sports, etc. are more prone to otomycosis. Usage of ear buds for cleaning the ear may traumatize the ear lining and may lead to secondary infection like otitis externa along with otomycosis. Long standing ear perforation with ear discharge may lead to development of fungal infection at times. At times, in advert use of antibiotic ear drops may also lead to secondary infection with fungus.

Presentation (Signs and Symptoms): Otomycosis presents with symptoms of pain, watery ear discharge, itching, decreased hearing and heaviness in the ear. It is accompanied with flakes of fungus in the discharge which may be blackish or white in colour. At times, on ear examination whitish fungus ball gives a camouflage appearance of the dull tympanic membrane. On cleaning with the suction, the fungus may be extracted and the actual ear drum or ear perforation may be seen.

Treatment: Ear cleaning with the suction or dry mopping should be done. Fungus should be cleaned to know the exact status of the ear drum. Antifungal ear drops like clotrimazole, miconazole are usually recommended in this situation. If the situation is more severe, oral antifungal agents like fluconazole should be used. The treatment may last up to 2-3 weeks depending upon the severity of the infection. In cases associated with otitis externa (infection in the outer ear), impregnated wick of icthymol glycerin is helpful in resolving the swelling and severe pain in the ear after cleaning the ear of the fungus. In ear perforation cases and in cases where normal ear drum is present, it is advisable to use antifungal ear drops to settle the ear discharge.

Prevention: Fungal infection in the ear can be prevented by not using antibiotic ear drops at random and without prescription. The antibiotic drops remove the good bacteria from the ear leading and making space for the secondary infection by the fungus. Apart from this, ear buds usage and instillation of oil should also be avoided.

Herpes Zoster Oticus (Ramsay Hunts yndrome)

Herpes is the infection caused by virus. It may involve different areas of the body and at times it may involve the ear and adjoining structures also. This virus has the tendency to affect a particular segment of the nerve. Another beauty of this virus is that it does not cross the midline. It is quiet clear from the way it spreads also since it moves along the nerve and normally a nerve also does not cross the midline.

Reasons: Herpes zoster infection occurs due to lower body immunity of the individual. This may happen due to various other infections in the body like HIV. Herpes zoster occurs in the elderly age group. Herpes zoster is also seen in individuals at later age that had chickenpox in the childhood.

Presentation (Signs and Symptoms): Herpes zoster Oticus presents with pain in the distribution of nerve segment of the facial nerve before the actual eruption of the blisters which are the hallmark of this infection.

Very severe pain along the facial nerve segment is seen in the individuals affected with this infection. Severe burning pain is followed by the eruption of vesicles and blisters along the distribution of the branch of the facial nerve. The vesicles are seen on the external ear, ear drum internally; face, on the inside of cheek and going up to the nose and rarely crossing the midline of face. Facial nerve palsy is also seen with the affected side looks like swollen. Severe to profound hearing loss may also be present along with spinning sensation in the head (Vertigo).

Treatment: Herpes zoster infection is difficult to diagnose in the beginning due to just presence of rash like presentation in the beginning which looks like some allergic reaction. At times it remains under diagnosed. The treatment consists of antiviral agents like Acyclovir, Valacyclovir. Pain is symptomatically controlled via analgesics. Local application of Acyclovir cream is used for facial vesicles and blisters. Artificial tears eye drops are used for eye involvement and to prevent corneal damage. Facial nerve physiotherapy is done to treat facial nerve paralysis.

Prevention: Vaccination for chickenpox in childhood may prevent the occurrence of Herpes zoster in elderly life. Healthy sex practices prevent development of AIDS which in turn prevents development of these types of dreadful infections in the individual.

Facial Nerve Palsy Trauma

Facial nerve has long and torturous route from the brain, on to the face and in the mouth. So it is prone to get involved in the infections and injuries of the head and neck section. Facial nerve moreover gets kinky in the ear section of the head and bound to get impacted via the injuries and infections in this region. Bell's palsy is the lower motor type of facial nerve disorder.

Reasons: Facial nerve involvement in the injuries and infections is not so uncommon. Facial nerve has a horizontal and vertical course in the ear and it comes out anterior to the ear and spread like tentacles on the face. Facial nerve palsy may occur due to idiopathic reasons where no obvious cause for the facial nerve palsy could be elicited. It may follow long standing history of ear discharge (unsafe Chronic Suppurative Otitis Media). Facial nerve may also be damaged via the surgeon while operating on the ear (Iatrogenic). During road side accidents, head injuries may involve fracture of the temporal bone leading to facial nerve injuries. Facial nerve may be involved in various infections of viral or bacterial etiology also.

Presentation (Signs and Symptoms): Facial nerve palsy presents with the symptoms of ear discharge, pain, fever, hearing loss and inability to drink or eat properly on affected side of face in cases with history of ear problems.

In cases of road side accidents, facial nerve palsy happens immediately after the incident in most of the cases. In these cases blood from the affected ear may come and facial muscles drooping on the affected side may happen.

Facial nerve paresis or palsy following ear surgery could be diagnosed then and there on the operating table with the affected side inability to close eyes and show teeth properly.

In most of the cases where no cause could be found, the patients show sudden involvement of facial muscles on affected side with inability to show teeth, drink water, brush properly, raise the eyebrows and fill air in the mouth.

Treatment: The treatment consists of ear surgery with immediate exploration of the facial nerve on the affected side in cases with ear discharge history. In cases of road side accident, it should be confirmed via CT scan or MRI that the nerve is damaged/transected and accordingly conservative or surgical approach should be considered. If the nerve is transected then it should be repaired at the earliest. The nerve in these cases may take 6-12 months for the recovery.

In other cases where no obvious cause could be found and with intact ear drum, treatment consists of antiviral therapy like Acyclovir along with steroids like dexamethasone and prednisolone. Along with that facial nerve physiotherapy is also recommended at the earliest generally on the day of diagnosis of facial nerve palsy. Facial nerve palsy of idiopathic cause takes about 3-4 weeks for the complete recovery.

Prevention: Facial nerve palsy in the ear discharging cases can be prevented by treating the ear disease at appropriate time. These cases should be operated so to prevent the spread of the infection to the facial nerve.

In the cases where the cause is unknown, prompt treatment and facial nerve physiotherapy prevent the occurrence of the any residual damage to the nerve. So in these cases, immediate treatment is again considered as important measure to prevent the complete damage to the facial nerve.

Trauma to the Ear

Ears are the structures which are important for hearing so probably that's why God has tried to save them from trauma in most of the cases of injury. Ear has cartilage so these don't get fractured. Most of the times, these get bruised.

Reasons: In today's mechanized world, accidents are common either on the road or in the industries. Trauma to the ears may happen due to marital violence or household fights. Slapping on the face and ears is common by the husband on to wife. Blunt trauma caused during such fights often result in ear perforation. Ear trauma may happen during fires in houses or factories. During road rage fights also, people may beat each other or even may bite the ear. As a feature of punishment also, in old times, ears or nose were chopped. At times, usage of ear buds has caused ear perforation while cleaning the ears. Crawling of the insects like cockroaches in the ears has also been associated with perforation of the ear drums. Trauma to the ear also occurs in the sports events like wrestling, cricket, boxing, judo, cycling, car race or martial arts. Trauma to the ear can be due to extreme hot or cold conditions also as while travelling in deserts or trekking on icy mountains.

Presentation (Signs and Symptoms): Ear trauma presents with pain in the ear, bleeding from the ear canal (in cases of ear perforation, head injury), bruises (in road side accidents) and hematoma in boxing or wrestling. In marital conflicts, usually the only symptom is heaviness in the ear and hearing loss. On examination, it is found to have ear perforation with ragged margins with slight blood in the ear canal.

Treatment: There is not much intervention in the initial period of the ear trauma cases. Most of these are treated conservatively and eventually most of them heal nicely. Ear perforations in marital conflicts heal in most of the cases if treatment is taken well in time. Road side accident injuries are treated with antiseptic dressings, antibiotics, analgesics, tetanus injections and surgery of the damaged ear, if required.

Prevention: Trauma to the ear could be prevented by using helmets while riding two wheelers, by using seat belts during car driving. Similarly during sports activities, head should be saved by using helmets. Ear perforation by ear buds, marital conflicts should be prevented from further damage by not instilling oil, ear drops and other home remedies but should be brought to the notice of the ENT specialist at the earliest.

Acute Tonsillitis

Tonsils are the structures in the throat which are the first line of defence in preventing infections occurrence in the throat. On opening mouth, they are seen to be located on the lateral walls of the throat, at the level of uvula (central hanging tissue seen with mouth open at the back of the throat). Tonsils are recognized by their rough surface in otherwise smooth contours of the mouth. Tonsils are an important tissue for preventing the development of infection in throat but in some people recurrent infections in the tonsils itself lead to embedment of infection in the core of the tonsils. In these cases even if no other source of infection is present from outside, the infection may flare up from the embedded bacterial infection from the tonsil itself. In such cases, it is recommended to remove the tonsils surgically.

Reasons: Tonsillitis is the bacterial infection; most commonly caused Beta- Hemolytic Streptococci, Staphylocci and/or Hemophilus influenza. Tonsillitis may happen with intake of cold drinks, sauce, spicy food, ice creams and refrigerated products in susceptible individuals. At times it happens with the change in the season from cold to warm and vice versa. Tonsillitis may happen because of diphtheria (thick membrane over the tonsils which bleed if tried to be removed), oral thrush (fungal infection), tuberculosis and various viral infections.

Presentation (Signs and Symptoms): These patients are mostly children and they present with complaint of throat pain, difficulty in deglutition, ear ache (in severe cases of tonsillitis), high grade fever with chills and rigors, cough, cold (if associated with adenoiditis). The pain is so severe in the throat that the patients are not able to swallow their own saliva also. There might be slight blood in the sputum on coughing which is due to severe congestion in the throat and not because of tuberculosis or cancer.

On throat examination, tonsils are severely congested with pus points over the tonsil. All the mucosal lining of the throat is reddish in colour. Pus points may also be seen in the posterior throat wall i.e. pharynx. On examination, neck lymph nodes are increased in size and they are tender on touch.

On ear examination, the ear drum is congested in varying degrees depending upon the extent of the infection reaching in the ear. It may be visible as congestion of only the central part of the tympanic membrane in the region of the handle of malleus to severe congestion of whole of the ear drum. At times, under the pressure of the fluid or pus in the ear, the ear drum may give way and ear drum perforation may happen with release of pus or blood from the ear drum.

Treatment: Acute tonsillitis is treated conservatively with broad spectrum antibiotics like cefpodoxime proxetil, azithromycin, cefuroxime axetil along with analgesics, anti allergics, anti pyretics, betadine gargles. In severe cases where swallowing of saliva is also difficult generally in childrens, patients are treated after admission in the hospital and are given intravenous antibiotics, analgesics and intravenous fluids and supplements.

Surgical removal of tonsils (tonsillectomy) is advocated where tonsillitis occurs more than 3 episodes per year and/or associated with complications like ear ache, ear discharge. Tonsillectomy prevents recurrent attacks of throat infection, improves growth of the children, increases height of the patient and prevents complications like ear perforation from happening.

Prevention: Tonsillitis prevention can be done by abstaining from taking cold refrigerated products, spicy food, sauce, various namkeens from the local shops. Doing warm saline gargles regularly also has preventive action. Sensitive persons should take care of proper clothing during change of weather which helps in preventing cough and cold. Children should preferably avoid taking cold refrigerated products immediately after coming from playing.

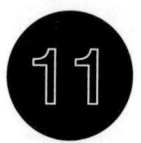

Dental Caries

Teeth are an integral part of the oral cavity. Teeth impart beauty and elegance to the person. Teeth are the hardest structure in the body and infection is difficult to penetrate through its enamel.

Reasons: Teeth do not catch the infection easily. But in today's world, these are the ones which are not taken care properly. Since early childhood, eating of candies, ice cream, chocolates, hot and cold liquids taken simultaneously spoil the hygiene of the teeth. Apart from this, irregular, improper teeth brushing habits take the sheen out of the teeth. Medications for the treatment of various infections could result in damage to the teeth in the form of staining, increasing brittleness and other disorders. Due to these, dental caries may set in at an early age.

Presentation (Signs and Symptoms): Patients with dental caries present with pain in the mouth and the pain radiating to the ear on the affected side. On examination, they have the infected tooth which has blackened and has reduced in size. There is adjacent swelling in the gums with the swelling of the affected lymph nodes in the neck. These lymph nodes are tender on touch and there temperature may be raised on palpation. Apparently ear drums have a normal look and are not congested in these cases.

Treatment: Dental caries is treated by removal of decayed material with filling of the defect by restorative materials like dental amalgam, porcelain. Root canal treatment or dental extraction is required in more damaged teeth. Use of broad spectrum antibiotics, analgesics, tooth paste and mouth wash is used to relieve the symptoms of pain and swelling in the gums and teeth. No active intervention is required for the pain relief of the ear since the treatment of the dental caries itself relieves the pain in the ear.

Prevention: Dental Caries can be prevented by regular brushing of the teeth, at least twice a day. Eating less of the candies, chocolates, sugar and sweets prevent the damage of the teeth. Scaling of the teeth at regular interval also prevent the occurrence of dental caries. Too hot and too cold at alternate times is damaging to the enamel and should be avoided. Soft brush should always be used for cleaning the teeth. Smoking, chewing tobacco, paan is injurious to the teeth and should be curtailed in day to day use.

Submandibular Lymphadenitis

The submandibular lymph nodes are the lymph nodes lying in close association of the submandibular gland. These lymph nodes are primarily associated with the lymphatic drainage of the oral cavity. At times, submandibular lymphadenitis is mistaken for submandibular gland infection.

Submandibular glands are the glands located at the level of angle of mandible in the floor of the mouth. These glands release saliva and helps in lubrication of the food eaten. The submandibular glands release saliva in conjunction with parotid and sublingual glands. The submandibular gland is commonly associated with calculi or stone formation in comparison to its peer group (i.e. sublingual and parotid gland).

Reasons: Submandibular lymph nodes are involved in the infections of the oral cavity and are commonly affected due to tonsillitis, pharyngitis, dental caries and carcinoma of oral cavity. Submandibular lymphadenitis is commonly seen in children with throat infections and submandibular lymph node involvement is common in the malignancy of the head and neck region in the elderly adults following smoking, chewing tobacco, etc.

Presentation (Signs and Symptoms): Submandibular lymphadenitis (inflammation of the lymph nodes following infection) presents with the complaint of pain in the submandibular region radiating to the ears, difficulty in swallowing, fever, pain throat. The children usually presents with the tender swelling in the region of submandibular lymph nodes with raised skin temperature locally. There might be some redness in that region also. Ear examination is usually normal without much of the findings.

Submandibular lymph nodes involvement in cancer of the oral cavity in elderly usually presents as a painless swelling without raised temperature in that region, with patient virtually having minimal symptoms of pain, fever, etc.

Treatment: Submandibular lymphadenitis is treated via regular broad spectrum antibiotics like azithromycin, cefpodoxime proxetil, cefadroxyl, etc. and analgesics. Betadine gargles with luke warm water is helpful in resolving the throat infection.

Submandibular lymph node involvement in malignancy is usually treated either by radiation or by radical neck dissection in conjunction with surgical excision of the cancer in the oral cavity.

Prevention: Submandibular lymphadenitis can be prevented by taking care of the throat by means of gargling with saline luke warm water. Avoidance of the food or cold drinks which can cause the throat infection in other way can prevent occurrence of this condition.

In adults, avoidance of smoking, chewing tobacco can prevent the occurrence of malignancy.

Barometric Trauma during Scuba Diving and Seafloor Walking

Scuba diving and sea floor walking involves the individual to go deep in the sea water for recreational or information collection purposes. It involves the diver to remain underwater for longer duration. Apart from fun and work, it has got its own problems associated and probably commoner is ear problem. Today this activity is becoming more and more common with increase in tourism and sporty attitude by the tourists, so the need for awareness for this problem is also very necessary to prevent oneself from the damage caused by this problem.

Reasons: Barometric trauma occurs due to sudden rise in the pressure in the middle ear during ascend after doing scuba diving and seafloor walking. The high pressure is transmitted through the eustachian tube in the middle ear leading to this condition. It may happen more commonly in patients already having acute nose and throat infections like pharyngitis, tonsillitis and sinusitis. Since in these patients, infection tend to travel much faster in the middle ear and cause barometric trauma.

Presentation (Signs and Symptoms): The usual symptoms of barometric trauma are heaviness in the ears, pain, decreased hearing, fullness in the ears and feeling of fluid coming out of the ear/s. If the pressure is too much, giddiness, nausea and vomiting feeling may also be noticed. On ear examination, the ear drum is congested with fluid levels. There is usually no perforation, though the ear drum is bulged out.

Treatment: Only conservative management with analgesics, mucolytic agents usually correct the condition. Valsalva manoeuvre is generally contraindicated since it may further raise the pressure inside the ear drum. Swallowing movements generally help in relieving the pressure in the ears either by drinking liquids, chewing gums or just doing it without actually drinking anything. Ear drops and warm oil instillation in the ears are contraindicated. Usually the condition takes 1-2 weeks to resolve.

Prevention: Adequate information to the diver about the safety measures during scuba diving and sea walking should be explained beforehand. They should be advised about the problems encountered after the activity. Any kind of valsalva manoeuvre should be avoided. As far as possible, calmness should be maintained after the person feels pressure, heaviness and fullness in the affected ear/s. Swallowing movements during ascend after scuba diving or sea floor walking helps in preventing the barometric trauma to occur since this keeps on balancing the increase in pressure in the middle ear. Also ascend should be slow and it should not be too fast so that the ears get the time to balance the pressure changes from sea floor to the surface.

Mumps

Parotid glands are the salivary glands which are situated in front of the ear and responsible for the secretion of saliva in association with the submandibular glands and the sublingual glands.

The saliva helps in mastication of the food by making it soft.

Mumps is the condition in which parotid glands are infected by the mumps virus.

Vaccination with MMR is routinely given in infants to prevent the development of mumps, measles and rubella.

Reasons: Mumps occurs due to the mumps virus which infiltrates the parotid gland/s and cause the swelling.

It is contagious and may spread to others through the use of common utensils, drinks contaminated by the saliva of the infected person.

It may spread to others via cold and cough in which droplet infection may cause the infection to others.

Presentation (Signs and Symptoms): Mumps present with the swelling of the parotid glands either unilaterally or bilaterally, on both sides more commonly along with fever, dryness of mouth, orchitis and pain in the ears.

Pain in the ears is not present in all the cases and is seen in only a few.

Difficulty in chewing or masticating food is due to less saliva produced.

On examination of the parotid region, in front of the ear, the parotid gland is tender to touch.

Treatment: Mumps is a self limiting infection mostly.

Treatment of mumps is only supportive, treated only with paracetamol and plenty of fluid intakes.

Antibiotics (cefpodoxime proxetil, azithromycin, cefuroxime axetil) are to be used if there is associated secondary infection of the mouth.

Citrus fruits should be avoided since they cause increased salivation leading to more pain in the mouth and ears.

Prevention: Mumps can be prevented by the vaccination of the infants in their early lives.

This infection can further be curtailed by avoiding contact with the infected individuals.

Washing of the hands with soap and water or using hand sanitizer helps in removing the germs.

Sharing of the same spoons, container and utensils should also be curtailed to minimize the infection spread.

Apthous Ulceration

Ulceration is the breach in the normal continuity of the mucosal layers in the alimentary canal.

Normally the lining of the mouth or elsewhere in the gastrointestinal system is in continuity and no break is seen. But at times, this break occurs resulting in apthous ulceration in the mouth.

Reasons: Apthous ulceration may occur due to various causes. In mouth, it could be due to recurrent tongue bite, dental caries, sharp denture, missing denture, chewing tobacco, alcohol intake, spicy food and smoking.

Apthous ulceration due to local infections like acute tonsillitis, pharyngitis, ludwig's angina, adenotonsillitis, sinusitis, etc.

In systemic causes, to name a few, it may due to generalized malnutrition, anemia, hepatitis, constipation, diarrhoea, diabetes, vomiting and carcinoma.

In prolonged high grade fever due to malaria, typhoid, gastroenteritis, dengue, viral fever, etc., apthous ulceration is seen.

At times, it may be due to overdose of medicines, antibiotics, analgesics, etc. by the treating physician.

Presentation (Signs and Symptoms): Apthous ulceration presents with pain in the mouth with difficulty in chewing and swallowing food and liquids, even at times their own saliva. The pain from mouth may radiate to the ear/s.

On examination of the mouth, tongue or other part of oral mucosa shows crater like lesion with reddish margins. The lesion may be single or multiple depending upon the severity of the disease. These may vary in size from few millimetres to few inches.

Treatment: Apthous ulcer treatment is usually conservative. It is commonly treated with Rebagen,

B-complex syrup or tablets along with mild analgesics like diclofenac, paracetamol, etc.

A local gargle with mild analgesic and anaesthetic agent like Tantum mouth wash is useful for the pain relief before meals. After meals gargles with Betadine is also effective in cleaning the ulcerated area of the microbes and residues of food particles.

Local application of Lexanox gel, Hexigel or Mucopain gel is effective in reducing the severity of the pain and healing of the ulcer.

Apart from this, specific treatment for the concurrent infection should also be carried on.

Prevention: Apthous ulceration could be prevented by treating the cause. For example, in dental caries or sharpness of the tooth, the tooth treatment should be started.

Recurrent teeth bite happens to be in over anxious personalities at time, so they should be advised to take their meals with patience. Otherwise also, meals should be taken with adequate time interval and should not be taken in haste.

Treatment of the systemic disorders with proper medicines will prevent the incidence of the apthous ulceration.

Non judicious usage of medicines should be avoided to prevent the occurrence of this problem.

Ludwig's Angina

Angina literal meaning is Strangling.

It should not be confused with Angina Pectoris or pain in the chest representing Heart Attack.

Ludwig's Angina is the infection in the Submandibular space.

The swelling in this region becomes so much that it causes compression of the airway leading to strangling like condition and hence its name of Ludwig's Angina (After the name of the Physician who first described this condition).

Reasons: The most common cause of Ludwig's Angina is the teeth infection (mostly molars) in the lower set of teeth.

The other uncommon causes may be injury in the submandibular region may be due to accidents, etc.

At times, capping of the molars after improper root canal treatment of the molar teeth makes it difficult to ascertain the cause of this infection.

Presentation (Signs and Symptoms): Ludwig's Angina is a life threatening condition if not handled appropriately at the right time.

It causes severe infection in the submandibular space leading to extensive swelling in the region with pain in the throat and neck.

Often the patient is unable to swallow his own saliva.

The pain may radiate to the ears.

The neck is also stiffened due to the infection. Fever with stridor is also present.

On oral examination, dental caries is present in the molars with swelling in the gums.

It may not be apparent on examination if the patient has undergone root canal treatment and is having cap on its top. But the positive history of the treatment for the caries tooth is present.

On examination of the submandibular region, note is made of the redness and board like, hardened skin of this region.

Drooling of the saliva from the mouth is present.

Treatment: Active management is required in these cases.

Immediate admission should be done in the hospital.

Incision and drainage of the submandibular region should be done at the earliest under general anaesthesia.

Maintenance of the airway should either be done via nasotracheal (passing airway tube from nose to the trachea) intubation or tracheostomy (making an opening in the windpipe), if required.

This should be done under proper Broad spectrum antibiotics, analgesics and other supportive treatment.

Regular antiseptic dressing with Betadine ointment or lotion should be done every day for few days followed by alternate days after sufficient recovery is obtained.

Dental treatment should be followed at the earliest after the recovery from Ludwig's angina.

Prevention: Dental caries should be treated appropriately to prevent the occurrence of this entity. Accidental injuries in the submandibular and sublingual area should be dealt at the earliest to prevent the spread of the infection and development of Ludwig's Angina.

Ornamental Piercing should be avoided in the region below the tongue, in the area of submandibular duct opening.

Malignant Otitis Externa

As the name suggests, it is not related with any malignancy but is the name given to the severe, progressive debilitating infection in the ear canal which is seen in Diabetics. Malignant otitis media is the necrotizing infection of the ear which spreads to involve the soft tissue around the ear and skull base, if care is not taken at right time.

Reasons: Malignant otitis externa is due to the uncontrolled diabetes in elderly patients wherein the infection ensues in the external ear following slight trauma, self ear cleaning, instillation of oil, etc.

It may be seen in immuno-compromised individuals like those who are on high doses of steroids, AIDS, Chemotherapy.

In most of the individuals, the causative agent is a bacterium named Pseudomonas aeruginosa.

Presentation (Signs and Symptoms): Pain in the ear canal is the hallmark of the symptoms in Malignant otitis externa.

Initially, it starts with minimal symptoms of otitis externa.

But as the disease progresses, it causes necrosis of the local tissue in the ear canal and spread to the Parotid gland, Temporo-mandibular joint and soft tissues at the skull base.

On examination, initial signs are swelling and redness in the ear canal extending to pinna.

The ear drum is usually intact.

Facial nerve involvement, hoarseness of the voice is seen later with the progression of the infection.

Treatment: Treatment of Malignant Otitis Media is with antibiotics and surgery.

Initially it should be started with Ciprofloxacin and if required debridement of the necrotic tissue should be done.

Antibiotic sensitivity should be done and if required injectables according to the sensitivity should be added.

Proper diabetic control, antibiotics and surgical debridement improves the outcome.

The progressive involvement of the Facial nerve (VIIth) and vagus nerve (Xth) are usually the grave signs in malignant otitis externa with poor prognosis.

Prevention: Strict maintenance of the diabetes control is very important to prevent the occurrence of this condition.

Ear trauma by any means should be avoided.

Prompt treatment and surgical intervention (if required) prevent the severe complications in this condition.

Foreign Bodies in the Ear

Ear canal is torturous and it has the narrowest portion (isthmus) at the junction of outer third to the inner $2/3^{rd}$ of the ear canal at the level of cartilage and bony junction of the ear canal.

Foreign bodies located lateral to the isthmus are more easily removable than the ones located medial to the isthmus.

Reasons: Foreign bodies in the ear invariably get lodged in the children while playing. This may be in the school or at home.

Most of the children are below 5 years of age.

These may be put in either by themselves or by their partners.

Mostly these are crayons, peas, cereals, steel balls, toy parts, thermocole, etc.

In adults, foreign bodies like match stick broken part, cockroaches, holi colour, insects like ant, mosquito, etc. are seen.

Recurrent insertion of foreign bodies in ear may be seen in mentally challenged children or adults.

Presentation (Signs and Symptoms): Foreign bodies in the ear present with the pain and blockage in the ear.

Usually in cases of children, the parents themselves give the positive history of insertion of foreign body by the child.

In adults, the similar complaints are present. In cases where live insects have gone in the ear, the patients give the crawling sensation, biting in the ear by the insect.

On examination, the foreign body is seen in the ear.

There may be perforation in the ear drum.

At times, very small foreign bodies like red ant are difficult to be visualized but the positive symptoms by the patient and proper visualization under microscope usually confirms the diagnosis. It might be found sticking to the ear drum and will show movement occasionally.

Prior trial of removal of the foreign body by the patient or by the general physician often increases the pain, bleeding in the ear with the impaction of the foreign body and difficulty in its removal especially in metallic and hard substance foreign body.

Treatment: Treatment is examination of the ear under microscope and removal of the foreign body.

At times when the foreign body is impacted, postaural route may be used to remove the foreign body. Antiseptic dressing of the ear is done with soframycin ointment which is normally removed after 2-3 days.

Antibiotics, pain killers are given according to the need.

Prevention: Small children should be under observation and they should not be allowed to play with the things which can act as a foreign body in the ear.

Adults while sleeping on the floor should cover their ears with a cloth or muffler or cap to protect themselves from the entry of mosquitoes or insects or cockroaches in the ears.

Impaction of the foreign body may happen if it will be tried by an inexpert for the removal.

Dermatitis of the External Ear

Allergic dermatitis is the skin disease with the development of rashes or maculo-papular lesion after coming in contact with the allergen.

In general, dermatitis of the external ear occurs in those individuals who are already predisposed to eczema.

It may be hereditary also.

Reasons: The ear skin may become sensitive and produce allergic reaction following the contact with the artificial jewellery (especially nickel containing ear rings or other jewellery), hair dyes, hair lotions, hair sprays, cosmetic creams, shampoos and hair conditioners.

Presentation (Signs and Symptoms): Dermatitis of the ear shows typical symptoms of itching, burning or pain in and around the ear.

Often there is severe irritation and on scratching, the lesions spread to adjoining areas.

Secondary infection may follow in these lesions if appropriate treatment is not taken on time.

On examination, vesicular lesions are seen around the ear with redness.

Scalding and dryness is often found.

Secondary infection cases show change of exudates from these lesions from serous to yellow (pus) and appearance of these lesions change from pale white to yellowish hue.

Treatment: Treatment of the lesions is with the use of anti-inflammatory, antibiotic impregnated, steroidal creams.

Aluminium acetate dressings (Burow's solutions) or Mupirocin with steroid ointment dressings are often helpful in resolving the infection.

1% hydrocortisone cream application is usually helpful in resolving the vesicular eruptions or serous exudates vesicles.

Itching can be reduced by oral anti-allergic agents like ebastine, loratadine, cetrizine, etc.

Prevention: Dermatitis of the ear can be prevented by avoiding the allergens which produce allergic reaction.

If a person is allergic to cosmetic cream, hair dyes, hair conditioner etc. then he should avoid the use of such substances.

Scratching or rubbing of the vesicles could lead to secondary infection so that should also be avoided to prevent the exaggeration of the infection.

Haematoma of the Auricle

Blood collection in ear is not uncommon.

It occurs following the rupture of the blood vessels in the external ear.

Blood gets collected between the cartilage and the perichondrium (the layer of soft tissue from where the nutrition goes into the cartilage).

This causes loss of blood supply to the cartilage.

It is non infective condition of the ear.

Reasons: Haematoma of the ear happens following injury or trauma.

It may be following boxing, wrestling, rugby football activities. In children it may happen due to child abuse.

Presentation (Signs and Symptoms): In acute phase, it usually presents with pain in the ear.

On examination, there is localized swelling of the pinna with loss of normal contours of the ear. The rest of the ear is normal looking without any redness or congestion or pain.

In long standing and untreated cases, the blood clot gets organized and causes permanent disfigurement with loss of normal contours of the ear. It is not painful on palpation or touching.

Treatment: Incision and drainage under strict asepsis is the ideal treatment.

Firm dressing should be applied following the surgery.

Repeated aspirations may be required in these cases.

Prevention: Usage of head mask is required while playing risky games like wrestling, football and rugby. Immediate attention to the injury and treatment prevents the development of cauliflower ear which is the name given to the deformed ear.

Osteoma of the External Auditory Canal

Bony protrusions are not uncommon in the body. Excessive bone formation activity leads to formation of osteomas.

These are not cancerous and only benign tumours.

These are localized swellings which don't have the tendency to spread to other areas.

Reasons: No definite reasons have been attributed to the development of the osteomas.

Ocean swimming and radiation may have some role in the development of osteomas.

Presentation (Signs and Symptoms): Osteomas mostly have not much of the signs and symptoms.

These are usually painless.

Osteomas are often diagnosed due to impacted wax with secondary infection resulting in the pain and blockage sensation in the ear.

On examination, osteomas are solitary and pedunculated structures in the ear canal. These are hard in consistency and do not move on instrumentation.

Treatment: Surgical excision of the osteoma is the treatment of choice.

Medical treatment does not have any role in this condition.

Since recurrence of the osteoma is common so repeat surgeries may be required in this condition.

Prevention: No absolute prevention protocol is there for the development of the osteomas.

But ocean swimming and radiation exposure should be avoided as far as possible in predisposed individuals.

Aural Polyps (Ear Canal Polyps)

Polyps are benign, soft tissue masses which develop following long term irritation due to infection, hypersensitivity to a particular substance.

Reasons: Ear polyps occur in the long standing cases of unsafe ear perforation cases with Cholesteatoma.

It may also occur in safe ear perforation cases with long term infected discharge.

These may also occur following infected and impacted wax over a prolonged period.

Ear polyps may develop due to foreign body in the ear over a long duration of time.

It may also occur in swimmers.

Presentation (Signs and Symptoms): Ear polyp cases present with bleeding or ear discharge, pain in the ear, decreased hearing and heaviness on the affected side.

Ear examination show soft, pale to reddish, fleshy growth in the ear canal.

These may be single or in cluster.

On instrumentation, the attachment of the ear polyps may be seen to the ear canal skin, tympanic membrane or the bone in the postero-superior perforation in unsafe ear perforation.

Treatment: Surgical removal of the ear polyp is the mainstay of the treatment in most of the cases.

In some cases of impacted wax with otitis externa with aural polyp, the cleaning of the ear followed by ear packing with mupirocin ointment gauze packing helps in resolution of the polyp without surgery.

At times, ichthymol glycerine may be used in the ear packing.

In cases of unsafe ear with cholesteatoma, surgeries with removal of the disease from the bone and ear polyp are done together.

In cases where ear polyp is seen to be attached to ear canal skin without ear perforation, simple excision with ear packing with antibiotic ointment gauze helps in resolution of the ear polyp.

Prevention: Treatment of the underlying cause prevents most of the ear polyp development.

Proper hygiene of the ear should be kept.

Treatment of the ear perforation and impacted wax should be done in time to prevent the development of aural polyps.

Foreign bodies should be dealt in time to prevent the occurrence of ear polyps.

Cholesteatoma

It is the benign condition in chronic cases of postero-superior ear drum perforation associated with the invasion of the ear canal skin lining (squamous epithelium) in the mastoid bone.

The skin lining of the ear canal slowly creeps in the mastoid bone and spread to involve adjacent structures.

It has local spread only and never spread to distant areas.

It is a benign condition and is not cancerous.

Reasons: The ear drum gets perforated following infections from recurrent tonsillitis, adenoiditis or sinusitis in children.

When these discharging ears are not treated or tonsil, adenoid or sinus problem is not corrected in time, some of these having hole in the postero-superior quadrant of the ear drum develop cholesteatoma. Cholesteatoma occurs in discharging ears with ear perforation lying in the postero-superior quadrant of the ear drum.

In chronic cases, the ear canal epithelium grows into the adjacent bone i.e. mastoid bone.

It's an insidious process and may spread to involve bony ossicles (malleus, incus, stapes – which helps in the hearing), meningis (protective layer of the brain), semicircular canals (helps in the balance of the body), lateral sinus, brain and facial nerve.

Presentation (Signs and Symptoms): The patients with cholesteatoma have foul smelling scanty ear discharge, hearing loss, heaviness in the ear, pain, fever or headache.

Depending upon the extent of the disease, these may have vertigo, imbalance due to semicircular canal involvement.

Meninges involvement may lead to meningitis with features of photophobia, severe headache, vomiting, high grade fever and imbalance.

Facial nerve involvement causes facial nerve paralysis or paresis. Brain abscess may also develop.

On examination of the ear, usually ear perforation is seen in the postero-superior quadrant of the ear drum.

Mastoid tenderness may also be seen, if the infection has spread to the outer layer of the mastoid process (periosteum).

Pressing of the tragus few times may induce nystagmus and vertigo in patients with infection in the lateral semicircular canal (Fistula test).

These are in general few tests and signs which may be found in patients with cholesteatoma.

Treatment: Surgery is the mainstay of the treatment of cholesteatoma.

Mastoid bone is opened and disease is cleared from the area involved. Fresh ear drum is laid and ossiculoplasty is done to improve the hearing.

Broad spectrum oral or intravenous antibiotics, analgesics, anti-allergic medicine and other supplements are also given to enhance the recovery.

Complications resulting as a result of spread of cholesteatoma are to be treated according to the set protocol for those conditions.

Prevention: Discharging ears should always be treated at the earliest.

In some of the patients; tonsillectomy, adenoidectomy or functional endoscopic sinus surgery may be required to prevent spread of the infection from these sites to the ear.

Acute Sinusitis

Sinuses are structures which are in association with the nose.

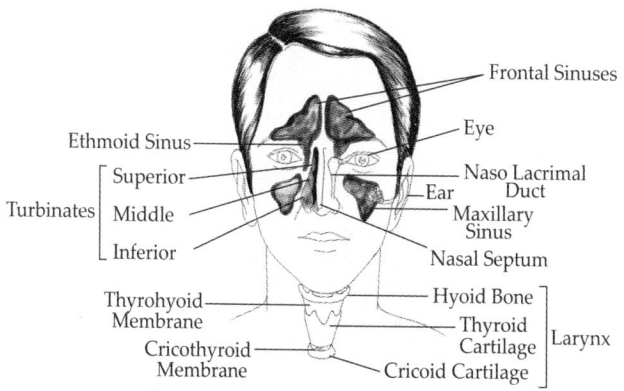

Fig. 3.1 Picture Showing Various Sinuses and Laryngeal Framework

These help in breathing, cleaning the inspired air of bacteria, pollutants, virus, etc., production of the mucus for humidification of the air, lightening the weight of the skull, imparts resonance to the voice, coolness to the eyes and the brain.

Sinuses have the importance of cleaning the sinuses by the mucociliary action.

Reasons: Infection of the sinus is common. These may be bacterial, viral, fungal or allergic.

Sinusitis may occur with sudden change in temperatures also.

Deviated nasal bone or other anatomical abnormalities may lead to decrease air flow resulting in growth of the organisms and thus precipitating sinusitis.

Allergic or infective pathologies may lead to development of the polyps (fluid filled pale whitish, thin membranous, grape-like structures) in the sinuses.

Infection in adenoid tissue in naso-pharyngeal area (the junction of nose and throat) may also contribute to sinusitis.

Foreign body in the nose for long period may mimic the symptoms of the disease.

Presentation (Signs and Symptoms): The patients of acute sinusitis present with symptoms of nasal congestion, nasal blockage, clear or muco-purulent nasal discharge, nasal bleeding at times, difficulty in breathing, headache, fever, watering of eyes, dry mouth.

Referred pain to the ear is indicated when the infection travels to ear.

Heaviness in the ears with decreased hearing, hearing voices in the ear is also associated complaints.

Pain to the ear is more often seen in the patients of acute sinusitis who have recently boarded a flight. On examination of the nose, the nasal cavity shows mucopurulent discharge, redness of the mucus membranes of the nose, congestion of nasal turbinates.

Mouth breathing will also be noted.

Puffiness around the eyes, pain on palpating maxillary and frontal sinuses may be elicited.

Treatment: Conservative management is the initial mode of treatment. Broad spectrum antibiotics, Anti-allergic, Analgesics are the medicines usually given for the treatment.

Surgical management with Septoplasty (Correction of deviation in nose septum) and Functional Endoscopic Sinus Surgery (FESS) are considered in recurrent cases of sinusitis.

CT scan should always be done before going ahead with the surgery to see the extent of the disease in the sinuses.

Prevention: Avoidance of the stuff which precipitates sinusitis should be curtailed.

Cold drinks, ice creams, cold water and in general refrigerated products should be avoided.

Abstinence of smoking helps in the prevention of sinusitis.

Carcinoma of the Ear (Pinna)

In General, Cancer at any place shows the proliferation of the cells at a rapid rate than the normal and their tendency to migrate to different regions and follow the similar growth pattern. This in turn hampers the working of that organ.

Carcinoma of the ear is slow growing cancer. It spreads to the adjoining structures at a very late stage where the individual does not give any care to the developing tumor.

Reasons: There is no obvious reason for the development of the carcinoma of the ear. It is usually seen in elderly individuals and not in the young people.

Presentation (Signs and Symptoms): Usually the cancer presents as an ulcerated, dry crusty or cystic lesion on the ear.

These are slow growing and take years to spread to the adjoining structures like parotid gland, mandible and other lymph nodes in the neck.

The patients normally take these lesions as dry crusts and keep on scratching on these lesions.

Pain in the ear is felt when the tumour spreads to the ear canal and middle ear.

Mild bleeding due to scratching may also be complained by the patients.

Treatment: Tumour is removed completely along with the adjoining normal skin margin (Wide excision) is the usual remedy for the cancer of the ear.

Radiotherapy may be required in cases with extensive spread.

Prevention: Scratching of the cancer lesion of the ear should be avoided to prevent spread of the cancer.

Crusting lesion of the ear should be promptly reported to the otolaryngologist so that adequate treatment will prevent its further extensive growth and extensive surgery.

Cerebellopontine Angle Tumour (Acoustic Neuroma)

In the brain, the nerve of hearing and balance (vestibulo-cochlear nerve or VIIIth cranial nerve) passes through the bony canal which is called internal auditory meatus. The tumour in this nerve begins in this canal.

The nerve has a long course before it innervates the cochlea and vestibule.

The tumour enlarges and presents in the region of cerebellum and pons, thus the name of cerebellopontine angle tumour.

It is slow growing tumour which has low propensity to migrate to other regions.

It mainly has problem because of the difficult approach to excise it and its tendency to recur.

Reasons: There's no known reason for the development of cerebellopontine angle tumor.

It is mainly seen in elderly females.

In modern era, the rate of cerebellopontine angle tumour has suddenly increased with the excessive usage of the mobile phones.

Presentation (Signs and Symptoms): The usual symptoms of acoustic tumour are deafness and tinnitus (ringing sensation or whistle like sensation in the ear).

The other symptoms due to enlargement of the acoustic neuroma are facial nerve weakness, improper gait and breathing difficulty.

The pain in the ear and in the region behind the ear is the referred pain from the compression of the nerve.

On examination, ear drums are normal in appearance.

On audiometry (computerized hearing test), moderate to severe sensori-neural hearing loss may be elicited.

MRI (magnetic resonance imaging) or CT (computerized tomography) can usually detect the lesion at the earliest, MRI being the investigation of choice.

Treatment: Once diagnosed, surgical excision is the treatment of choice.

Radiotherapy may be required post surgery for the eliminating the residual tumour.

Oral antibiotics and other supplements do not have much role in the management of the acoustic neuroma.

Prevention: Limited usage of mobile phones may be helpful in the prevention of Acoustic Neuroma. Tinnitus, deafness and headache symptoms should be dealt carefully in all the patients so that early detection of the tumour may prevent extensive complications.

Quinsy

Tonsil is an important tissue in the oral cavity for preventing the entry of infection to the throat and chest.

Since it does not have a capsule so the infection from the mouth may enter its crypts and remain embedded for long giving rise to recurrent tonsillitis in susceptible individuals.

Tonsil removal is required in patients who have 3 or more episodes of tonsillitis per year.

Tonsil infection when extends from its capsule to the adjoining tissue (peritonsillar region) then it is called Quinsy. It may extend to involve the soft palate and uvula also.

Reasons: Infection in the tonsil may spread to the adjacent soft tissue and cause peritonsillar abscess (Quinsy).

Tonsil infection may happen due to bacteria, virus or fungus.

It may also occur in susceptible individuals with change in weather.

Presentation (Signs and Symptoms): Quinsy presents with difficulty in swallowing, severe pain in the throat, hot potato voice, fever, dribbling of saliva from the side of mouth and pain in the ear. Pain in the throat is usually unilateral.

On examination of the throat, the tonsils are usually congested and pus extruding from the tonsils. The affected side show large swelling above the tonsillar region, displacing the uvula on the other side. The globular swelling can readily be identified since it looks quite obvious on oral examination. It stands out with yellowish centre with adjoining reddish area as is observed in a pus filled structure.

The lymph nodes in the neck are also enlarged and tender on palpation, more on the side of peritonsillar abscess.

Treatment: Quinsy is normally treated by incision and drainage of the abscess. The incision is usually given in the most dependent and prominent part of the abscess.

Drainage is followed by rigorous course of broad spectrum antibiotics (cefpodoxime proxetil, azithromycin, cefuroxime axetil), analgesics, betadine gargles and other supplements.

Hospitalization is mandatory to carry out this treatment.

Prevention: Quinsy can be prevented by taking adequate care and treatment when tonsillitis develops. Since it extends to the adjacent tissue after tonsillitis, so all precautions taken to prevent tonsillitis should be followed.

Cold refrigerated products, spicy, saucy food should be avoided along with curtailing smoking. Tonsillectomy should be done in the patients having recurrent tonsillitis.

Regular warm saline or betadine gargles also help.

Retropharyngeal Abscess

Normally pharynx is the pinkish-red, velvety, wall-carpet like area seen at the back of the throat on oral examination.

Retropharynx is the area lying behind the pharynx and in front of the prevertebral space.

Reasons: Retropharyngeal abscess is seen in infants.

It is caused by the bacterial infections.

In adults, common cause of retropharyngeal abscess is tuberculosis of the cervical spine.

Presentation (Signs and Symptoms): Retropharyngeal abscess presents as painful swelling in the throat with difficulty in deglutition.

Pain is referred to the ear and head.

High fever, sore throat, respiratory distress is other associated symptoms.

On examination of the throat, abscess is seen abutting the soft palate. Posterior pharyngeal wall (posterior wall of the throat) is seen to be pushed anteriorly forward with severe congestion present in the pharynx.

Treatment: In infants and children, incision and drainage of the abscess is done from the throat.

In adults, anti-tuberculosis medicines are started along with incision and drainage of the abscess from the neck.

Prevention: Healthy diet, good sanitation environment is required to prevent the development of the disease.

Acute Cervical Lymphadenitis

Cervical lymph nodes are glands located in the neck region associated with the drainage of lymph from various lymphatic organs.

Lymph nodes have white blood cells, histiocytes and macrophages which help in killing bacteria, viruses and other infectious agents.

These basically act as filtering regions in the body where blood or lymph is cleared of the infectious agents and phagocytosis takes place by the white blood cells or macrophages.

Reasons: Cervical lymph nodes get inflamed due to infections in the neck region especially tonsils, submandibular glands, adenoids, parotid glands and sinuses.

Infection from tonsils etc. travel to these lymph nodes and in the process of clearance of the infectious organisms, these glands gets enlarged.

Presentation (Signs and Symptoms): The patients with acute cervical lymphadenitis presents with pain in the neck, fever, earache and symptoms pertaining to tonsillitis, parotid gland infection or sinusitis. Pain to the ear is often referred pain from the lymph nodes involved.

In tonsillitis, the patients may have additional cough and cold with difficulty in swallowing.

In parotid gland infection, pain associated with mastication of food may be an associated symptom.

In sinusitis, nasal blockage and cold are usually present.

On examination of the neck, the lymph nodes are usually enlarged, tender on touch, with raised temperature of the surface of the lymph node area in comparison of the rest of the neck.

The other signs pertaining to the region involved are usually present.

Treatment: Treatment for acute cervical lymphadenitis is generally conservative.

Broad spectrum antibiotics, pain killers and local treatment according to the area involved is given.

It usually takes one to two weeks for the resolution of the signs and symptoms of the disease.

Prevention: Abstaining from the cold refrigerated products, sauce and junk food should be advocated, in order to prevent from throat and nose infections which eventually lead to acute cervical lymphadenitis.

Diphtheria

Diphtheria is infection of the throat seen in children.

It is caused by the Cornybacterium diphtheriae, Gram Negative bacteria.

It may be life threatening in early childhood due to formation of a pseudo membrane on the tonsils, throat and larynx which eventually lead to obstruction of the airway.

It may be prevented by usage of DPT vaccine.

In Developed Nations, like USA and Canada, this infection is virtually nonexistent at present with vaccination of the children with Diphtheria vaccine.

Reasons: Diphtheria is mainly seen in young children, mostly in the age group of 2-3 years, in developing or under developed nations.

It is caused by the bacteria which may spread from one person to another by coughing and by nose and throat secretions.

Poor hygiene, pollution, malnutrition, improper sanitation and vaccination are the main reasons for its presence in the under developed nations.

Presentation (Signs and Symptoms): Young child usually presents with sore throat, fever, cough and difficulty in deglutition and at times referred pain in the ears.

On examination of the throat, tonsils are congested with false membrane formation on the tonsils, soft palate and posterior pharyngeal wall. It may involve the nose with smelly and blood stained discharge. The larynx and trachea may be involved leading to difficulty in breathing.

False membrane characteristically is greyish to brown in colour, firmly adherent to the surface and bleeds on removal from tonsil or other region and forms again after it is removed.

The cervical lymph nodes are enlarged and extremely tender on palpation.

Ear examination is more or less devoid of any characteristic signs.

Treatment: Conservative management with antibiotics like penicillin, erythromycin is the mainstay of the treatment.

Analgesics, nutritional supplements, Betadine gargles and diphtheria antitoxin are additional requirements.

Tracheostomy (Making hole in the Wind pipe and putting tracheostomy tube for maintaining airway) may be required in life threatening cases.

Prevention: Diphtheria can be prevented by proper vaccination with Diphtheria vaccine in early childhood.

Early treatment of Diphtheria with proper antibiotics and supportive treatment helps in preventing life threatening complications like respiratory distress, myocarditis (inflammation of heart muscles) and neuropathy.

Iatrogenic

Iatrogenic means condition developed due to the treatment by a physician.

In this particular context, the ear pain develops during the treatment by the ENT specialist.

A doctor will never try to cause the problem but mishappening during the treatment may result in ear pain.

Reasons: Iatrogenic ear pain may occur while cleaning the wax or fungus from the ear.

Ear perforation may happen while ear cleaning via syringing or ear probe cleaning.

Acute otitis externa may develop after syringing with unsterile water.

Bleeding from the ear may follow hard wax removal from the ear.

Foreign bodies may be pushed inside and may get impacted with improper technique.

Ear pain and perforation may follow the insertion of grommet (ventilation tube) in the intact ear drum. While cutting the residual pack in Otitis externa following the ear packing, the accidental cut may be done to the tragus.

Stitch removal may also lead to injury and infection of the ear pinna.

Facial nerve injury may occur during mastoid surgery leading to facial nerve paralysis and ear pain.

Presentation (Signs and Symptoms): Iatrogenic ear pain follows the procedure conducted by the physician.

Immediately during or after the procedure, the patient will have excruciating pain in the ear.

There may be associated symptoms of facial nerve paralysis if facial nerve is damaged during the mastoid surgery.

On examination of the ear, bleeding may be seen following wax removal or ear perforation. The foreign body may be impacted inside the ear with the blood all around.

Treatment: Ear perforation following Ear cleaning may heal well with conservative management and proper assurance to the patient and their attendants.

Impacted foreign body may be managed by conducting the procedure under general anaesthesia.

Ear perforation following grommet extrusion may involve the myringoplasty (new ear drum grafting).

Facial nerve exploration may be required in cases of facial nerve paralysis.

Prevention: For any procedure to be done by a physician, proper care and appropriate environment with good operation theatre facilities should be available.

Ear being a sensitive and important organ in the body, due care should be taken before going ahead with any procedure.

Otosclerosis

Otosclerosis is the condition in the ear where the stapes (bone involved in hearing) gets immobilized by the spongy new bone formation leading to conductive hearing loss.

Spongy new bone formation occurs in the region of promontory, near the oval window.

It occurs more commonly in middle aged female and may be hereditary in nature.

Reasons: Otosclerosis is hereditary in nature and occurs due to new spongy bone formation near the region of oval window where stapes is situated.

Ankylosis of the stapes leads to inability of the sound waves to be conducted to the inner ear for hearing thus leading to hearing loss.

Pregnancy, accidents and puberty commencement may predispose the patient to develop Otosclerosis.

Presentation (Signs and Symptoms): The patients with otosclerosis presents with bilateral gradual increasing conductive hearing loss, tinnitus (sounds like hissing, roaring, machine, pulsatile) and vertigo. The patient also suggests of better hearing in the presence of noise like motor car, near machines, etc. (Paracusis Willisii).

Ear pain is seen in few patients where the disease has advanced.

On examination of the ear, the tympanic membrane is normal in most of the individuals. In some, flamingo flush appearance of ear drum (Schwartze sign) is seen.

Audiometry shows conductive hearing loss which on repeated intervals show downward curve.

Treatment: Conservative management with Fluroide therapy may be considered in initial period. Hearing aid may be advisable in few who don't wish to undergo surgery.

Stapedectomy is the treatment of choice in these patients.

Prevention: Since it's the disease of hereditary nature, no preventive measures really works.

Glomus Tumours

Glomus tumours arise from glomus bodies present either on the jugular vein (blood vessel in the floor of the middle ear) or promontory (Prominent part of Cochlea, hearing organ). Glomus tumors are benign tumours and are not malignant.

There are two types of tumours-1. Glomus Jugularae, 2. Glomus Tympanicum.

Reasons: Glomus Tumours arise in the middle ear and spread in the temporal bone or in the middle ear cavity. Glomus Jugularae is more extensive and locally aggressive whereas Glomus Tympanicum is inactive and slow growing.

Presentation (Signs and Symptoms): Glomus tumours present with tinntus (voices which are heard with each pulse in the body i.e. pulsatile), heaviness in the ear, blood stained ear discharge, pain in the ear and decreased hearing.

Glomus Tympanicum presents as a middle ear polyp and may come in the external ear after perforating the ear drum.

Similarly, Glomus Jugularae presents as middle ear polyp but has more rapid spread in the adjoining area involving IXth, X, XI Cranial nerves. Further upward spread may involve facial nerve leading to facial nerve paralysis. The tumour may perforate the ear also.

On examination of the ear, initially a red mass may be seen in the floor of the middle ear cavity behind the intact ear drum.

If the ear drum is already perforated by the tumour, reddish mass is seen in the external ear canal which bleeds on probing.

Other cranial nerves IX, X, XI and VII may be involved depending upon extent of the tumour.

Treatment: Surgical removal is the mainstay of the treatment.

Glomus Tympanicum is more easily excised whereas Glomus Jugularae requires more extensive surgery.

Prevention: There is no preventive measure for this condition.

Carcinoma of the External Auditory Canal and Middle Ear

Cancer of the external auditory canal and middle ear is extremely uncommon.

Squamous cell carcinoma is the most common cancer found in the external auditory canal and middle ear. It is slow growing tumour.

Reasons: Carcinoma of the external ear canal and middle ear has been found to be associated with ear discharge over a prolonged period.

Trauma, frostbite, radiotherapy, psoriasis and actinic rays have also been instrumental in the development of the cancer of the external auditory canal and middle ear.

Chronic otitis externa and Marjolin's ulcer may again be linked to this cancer.

Presentation (Signs and Symptoms): The patients with cancer of the external auditory canal and middle ear tend to have severe, deep seated ear ache.

They have blood stained ear discharge of recent onset after having purulent or muco-purulent ear discharge over the years.

Hearing loss, unsteadiness, facial nerve paralysis may also be present.

Parotid gland and IX, X, XI, XII cranial nerves involvement may be seen in late stages.

On examination of the ear, the blood stained discharge may be seen in the external meatus from the perforated ear drum. Swelling is seen in the external ear canal and middle ear.

CT scan or MRI is helpful in diagnosis and extent of the cancer.

Hearing test like audiometry will confirm the hearing loss.

Facial nerve damage will be characterized by inability to frown on the affected side along with inability to show teeth, incomplete closure of the affected eye, dribbling of saliva and inability to fill air in mouth. The four cranial nerve involvement is shown by hoarseness, difficulty in swallowing and aspiration of the food or liquids while swallowing.

Treatment: Surgical removal of the tumour followed by radiotherapy is the treatment of choice in the carcinoma of the external auditory canal and middle ear.

Medical therapy does not have any role in this condition.

Prevention: Chronic ear discharge should be treated in time to prevent the development of this condition.

Crusting lesions of the external ear or pinna should be dealt appropriately.

Sun exposure should not be for prolonged durations.

Elongated Styloid Process (Eagles Syndrome)

Styloid process is the part of the temporal bone which is elongated, conical projection, lies just below the ear and serves attachment for various muscles. Its length may vary and at times it may be elongated up to the bed of tonsil.

Reasons: Styloid process may be elongated as a part of normal development and it does not have any particular reason for elongation.

At times, it may be fractured after an accident and resulting granulation tissue around the fractured segment may lead to development of symptoms.

Presentation (Signs and Symptoms): Elongated Styloid process present with the symptoms of pain in the mouth while eating, pain while swallowing, pain on changing head positions, cervical pain, foreign body sensation in the throat, changes in voice, headaches, dizziness and ear pain.

On examination, there may be swelling of one of the tonsil on the affected site or there may be no apparent sign of elongated styloid process.

On palpation of the tonsillar region, the tip of the styloid process can be felt.

X-rays or CT scan may be helpful in clinching the diagnosis.

Treatment: Conservative management may involve usage of analgesics.

Surgical removal may involve tonsillectomy and excision of part of the styloid process.

Prevention: No obvious way of protecting oneself from elongated styloid process.

Glossopharyngeal Neuralgia

Glossopharyngeal nerve is the IXth Cranial Nerve which innervates the tongue (Glosso-) and the throat (Pharynx).

Apart from this, it has various other nerve branches supplying stylopharyngeus muscle, skin of the outer ear and other organs of the body.

Glossopharyngeal neuralgia is more common after the age of 40 years.

Glossopharyngeal neuralgia is the condition characterized by severe pain in the tongue, back of nose and ears lasting from few seconds to few minutes.

Reasons: In most of the cases of Glossopharyngeal neuralgia, the cause could not be diagnosed.

But in some, Glossopharyngeal neuralgia may occur due to throat and nose infections.

It may occur due to tumours arising in the base of the skull.

If any blood vessel is impinging upon it, then even this condition may precipitate.

Presentation (Signs and Symptoms): Glossopharyngeal neuralgia presents with severe pain along its sensory innervations.

The severe pain is perceived in the back of the throat, tongue, posterior part of nose and in the ear.

The pain is usually unilateral and the patient is in severe agony.

The pain in this condition may be triggered by talking, chewing, coughing or swallowing.

On examination of the patient with glossopharyngeal neuralgia, in most of the cases no obvious sign is elicited.

Ear, nose and throat examination is more or less normal.

In few cases, sinusitis or tonsillitis may be detected.

CT scan or MRI may show presence of the tumour pressing upon the nerve, if any malignancy is present.

Treatment: Conservative management consists of pain killers like paracetamol, diclofenac sodium, Carbamazepine, gabapentin and phenytoin are the most effective pain killers in this condition.

Since the pain is not controlled by simple analgesics, antidepressants are often added.

Antibiotics as per requirement of nose and throat infections may be initiated.

The intractable pain may be controlled by surgery i.e. the glossopharyngeal nerve is cut (rhizotomy). This is often effective in controlling the pain.

Prevention: Glossopharyngeal neuralgia may be prevented in few cases where sinusitis and tonsillitis are responsible by adequate treatment of the disease.

In most of the other cases where no cause could be elicited for this condition, no particular preventive measure is effective.

Infection in the Preauricular Sinus

Preauricular sinus is the congenital anomaly where a small opening is seen in front of the auricle, on the lobule, ascending limb of helix or tragus.

These sinuses have a blind end going in the external auditory canal.

At times, the sinus length may go upto the facial nerve also.

Preauricular sinus is often undiagnosed at the time of birth. These come to light when they get infected and lead to pain and swelling near the ear.

Reasons: Preauricular sinus is a congenital malformation and happens due to incomplete fusion of the first and second branchial arches during the time of embryogenesis.

Presentation (Signs and Symptoms): Preauricular sinus usually doesn't have any symptoms.

Sometimes in asymptomatic patients history of whitish material discharge through the sinus is present.

The signs and symptoms start with the infection in the sinus.

That leads to swelling, congestion and accumulation of the pus in the tract.

Patients complain of pain in and around the ear. Children may develop fever.

The purulent discharge is seen from the opening of the preauricular sinus.

Treatment: Excision of the whole preauricular sinus tract is the treatment of choice.

In acute stage, the infection is initially settled by broad spectrum antibiotics like cefpodoxime axetil, cefpodoxime proxetil, azithromycin, etc.

Analgesics like paracetamol, diclofenac sodium may also be required to be given.

Local application like mupirocin or betadine ointment can be used to cure the infection.

Incision and drainage of the infected preauricular sinus in acute stage is avoided as far as possible so that future excision of the sinus tract will be easier. Treatment is usually carried for 1 to 2 weeks.

Prevention: Since the preauricular sinus is a congenital malformation so none of the preventive methods are available for this condition.

Torticollis

Torticollis (Stiff Neck) is the condition where the neck gets stiffened due to spasm in the sternocleidomastoid or trapezius muscle. This condition is also called as 'Wry Neck'.

It can be congenital (since Birth) or Acquired (Develop in normal individuals in later part of life due to the damage to the muscle or nerve) in nature.

Torticollis is a painful condition characterized by rotation of the face and lateral bending of the neck.

Reasons: Congenital torticollis is due to birth trauma or malrotation of the foetus during pregnancy.

At times, it is not apparent at birth but gradually develops as is seen in some having family history of this disorder.

In some of the cases the cause of congenital torticollis is not clear.

Acquired torticollis may occur due to trauma to the neck, infections like tonsillitis, adenoiditis, retropharyngeal abscess, tuberculosis cervical spine, tumours or drug abuse.

Presentation (Signs and Symptoms): Patients with acute torticollis presents with pain in the neck, headache, neck stiffness, head tremor and ear pain.

Classically on examination, the neck is tilted on the side of torticollis and head is rotated on the opposite side.

The sternocleidomastoid and/or trapezius muscle on the affected side is taught and seems to stand out on physical examination.

On palpation, any neck movement on the opposite side is painful.

Facial asymmetry may be noted in the long standing cases and especially in congenital torticollis.

Ear examination is usually normal.

Throat examination may show the presence of tonsillitis or adenoid hypertrophy in affected cases.

Treatment: Conservative management of torticollis is done with hot fomentation, physiotherapy, neck exercises, analgesics (pain killers) and local application of ointment, gels like volini gel, relaxyl ointment, voveran gel, etc.

Surgery consisting of surgical release of the affected muscle is required in the cases not cured by the conservative management.

In congenital cases of torticollis, head position should be corrected before the age of 18 years to prevent the permanent disfigurement of the face.

Prevention: Torticollis can be prevented by proper delivery practice at the time of delivery of the baby. Tonsils, adenoids, cervical lymph nodes, retropharyngeal abscess, tuberculosis cervical spine should be treated in time to prevent the development of torticollis.

Surgery in the neck region should be done with adequate care so to prevent iatrogenic development of torticollis.

Cerebellar or neck tumours should be dealt at the earliest to prevent such complications to happen.

Temporo-mandibular Joint Syndrome

TMJ (Temporo-Mandibular Joint) joins the lower jaw to the skull.

Temporo-mandibular joint is the joint which helps in mastication of the food in the mouth, for speech and facial expressions.

This joint also helps in the opening and closure of the mouth.

Temporo-mandibular joint disorder may lead to the pain while chewing or difficulty in opening and closure of mouth.

Reasons: Temporo-mandibular Joint syndrome or disorder may occur due to arthritis, connective tissue disorder, trauma to the face or head, jaw clenching in the night, bruxism, aggressive personality with tendency to clinch mouth often, excessive tobacco chewing, smoking, degenerative changes in the joint with the age, hereditary conditions such as hypoplastic condyle of mandible.

Psychological stress leading to excessive grinding of the jaws may also lead to the development of this disorder.

Presentation (Signs and Symptoms): Symptoms seen in patients with the disorder of Temporo-mandibular joint are difficulty in chewing food, pain in the muscles of mastication often dull pain is perceived.

Pain may also be radiaed to the jaw and ear which gets bad with chewing, opening or closure of mouth.

Pain in the head, neck and shoulders may also be noticed in some patients.

Facial trauma history resulting in TMJ syndrome will be present in those patients who met an accident or got injured in the fight.

The jaw may get locked when the mouth is tried to be opened as may be seen in patients with this disorder.

On examination of these patients, the muscles of the mouth may be stiff on palpation.

The jaw opening is limited (Normal range is about 40 mm in adults from upper to lower anterior teeth) and unilateral facial swelling may be observed.

On palpation of Temporo-mandibular joint, the patient may show extreme pain on opening or closing of the mouth or with sliding movements of the joint.

Clenching or grinding of the teeth may also be noted on observation in these patients while they are sitting in the clinic.

Treatment: Hot fomentation and physiotherapy is the initial conservative treatment.

Analgesics and muscle relaxants may be required in chronic patients.

Antipsychotics or anti-depressants may be required in the ones with mental disorders leading to Temporo-mandibular syndrome.

Steroid injection in the Temporo-Mandibular joint may be required to be given in a few with severe symptoms.

Surgical management may be required where conservative management fails.

Prevention: TMJ syndrome patients need these preventive measures to control the development of this disorder.

Grinding or clenching of the teeth should be avoided as far as possible.

Psychotherapy for relaxation of the body, yoga or meditation may be required in those with aggressive behaviour or unstable personalities.

Regular hot massage of the facial muscles or face helps in curtailing the development of symptoms in this disorder.

Hard food or substances should be avoided and soft meals should be encouraged to prevent TMJ syndrome.

Neck and facial exercises involving temporomandibular joint area should be done.

Cancer of Larynx

Larynx or voice box is the voice producing organ of the body.

It is situated in the neck.

Vocal cords movement helps in the phonation.

Any infection or malignancy affects the vocal cords resulting in the change of voice or aphonia (complete loss of voice).

Cancer of larynx is more common in the males and it may be supraglottic (above the vocal cords), glottic (at the level of vocal cords) or subglottic (below the vocal cords) variety.

The tumor which is present at all levels i.e. supraglottis, glottis and subglottic is called Transglottic.

Most of the times, it is squamous cell carcinoma variety type on histopathology.

Reasons: Cancer of larynx is mostly seen in smokers.

At times, no obvious reason is present and the cause is idiopathic.

Presentation (Signs and Symptoms): Mostly these patients present with the complaint of hoarseness of voice, dysphagia, swelling in the neck and respiratory distress.

Ear pain is present in few patients which is usually the referred pain.

In few patients of supraglottic cancer, there may not be any presenting symptoms like change of voice or swelling in the neck. These cancers are diagnosed just by chance on routine examination.

On examination, the patient may show presence of swelling of neck on affected side due to lymph node spread of malignancy.

Otherwise there may not be any obvious features of malignancy on inspection of neck.

On palpation of the neck, the lymph nodes may be palpable and crepitus may be absent on movement of larynx from side to side (Normally a grating sound is produced on movement of larynx from side to side in normal individuals).

On laryngeal examination with indirect laryngoscopy or now a days with 70 degree endoscope, the fulgurating mass or cancer may be seen involving different regions of the larynx i.e. supraglottic, glottic or subglottic.

Confirmation of the cancer is done by taking biopsy of the lesion via direct laryngoscopy under anaesthesia.

CT scan is required to see the spread of the cancer in the adjoining areas.

Treatment: Cancer of the larynx is treated either by surgery or conservatively by radiotherapy.

Small lesions can be treated by radiotherapy alone.

Large tumours require surgical management with en bloc dissection and radical neck dissection of the lymph nodes followed by radiotherapy postoperatively.

In today's time, the treatment of cancer larynx is very effective in clearing the cancer and decreasing the mortality rate.

Modernization in the field of surgery and radiotherapy has significantly reduced the morbidity and mortality rate associated with carcinoma larynx.

Prevention: Smoking is closely associated with the development of carcinoma larynx, so it should be stopped or curtailed to prevent its occurrence.

Any hoarseness of voice or dysphagia should be properly assessed to rule out cancer since early detection of the cancer is always associated with better outcome.

Treatment of the cancer should be started at the earliest without falling prey to superstitious measures to prevent the complications due to delayed treatment.

Goitre

Thyroid gland is situated in the neck below the larynx.

It is a bilobed, butterfly shaped gland which lies upon trachea (the windpipe) at the level of cricoid cartilage.

Normally in the neck the thyroid gland is not seen on inspection and if it is visible that shows some type of goitre is present.

Thyroid gland maintains the basal metabolic rate, temperature in the body by secreting hormone like thyroxin. Calcitonin is another hormone produced by the thyroid gland which maintains the calcium homeostasis in the body.

Weight loss or weight gain may happen due to increase (hyper) or decreased (hypo) secretion of thyroxin hormone in the body, usually seen in females.

Reasons: Goitre is the condition in which the thyroid gland gets enlarged and is quite apparent on inspection.

It may be caused by the iodine deficiency, autoimmune disorders and malignancy.

It is common in hilly regions where iodine content in the soil is low.

Other reasons may be sarcoidosis, pituitary dysfunction and medications.

Presentation (Signs and Symptoms): Goitre may be detected present with the swelling in the neck. It may cause difficulty in swallowing and respiratory distress due to compression of underlying trachea and food pipe with increased size.

Pain in the ears may occur due to the stretching of the nerves due to enlarged size of the thyroid and is generally referred pain.

In Hypothyroidism, patient may have weight gain, hoarseness of voice, irregularity in menses, cold intolerance, mood swings.

Hyperthyroid patients have symptoms including palpitations, heat intolerance, nervousness, warm wet hands, breathlessness, tiredness and fine hand tremors.

On examination, the gland is enlarged on inspection and moves with the deglutition movement in the neck.

On palpation, thyroid lobes may be enlarged on one side or on both sides.

Further evaluation by laboratory tests (thyroid profile), thyroid scan, ultrasound of the thyroid gland, fine needle aspiration cytology and CT scan of the neck helps in diagnosing the cause of the goitre.

Treatment: Conservative management is the mainstay of the treatment in goitre till it enlarges to the extent that it compresses the airway or food pipe or it is malignant in nature.

Most of the Goitre patients are euthyroid (normal thyroid functioning) and do not need any medications.

Hypothyroid patients are treated with levothyroxine (thyronorm, Eltroxin) tablets and calcium supplements (Shelcal, Alfacalcidol, etc.).

Hyperthyroidism is treated with propylthiouracil, methimazol and radioactive iodine-131.

Goitre which is compressing the airway or foodpipe should be treated surgically and enlarged portion of the gland should be excised. This invariably leads to hypothyroidism which is corrected with levothyroxine supplement (thyroid hormone tablet) throughout life.

If malignancy is detected then it should be treated with anti-cancer agents (Radioactive iodine-131) along with surgical removal of the gland (thyroidectomy, lobectomy, etc.). Post operatively in malignancy patient's, radiotherapy may be required along with radioactive iodine-131 for complete ablation of the tumour.

Prevention: Goitre in endemic regions may be prevented by providing iodized salt.

If hypothyroidism develops in pregnancy (as is commonly seen) then immediate treatment should be started to prevent any damage to the developing foetus.

Cervical Spondylosis

Cervical spondylosis is the term used for wear and tear of the bones and joints (degenerative changes) of the cervical vertebrae which occurs with the aging process.

Spinal cord in the neck region passes through the cervical vertebrae and thus is protected by it.

The nerves to the neck, shoulder, upper limbs and part of the lower limbs pass through the cervical vertebral column.

These nerves may get compressed due to various reasons leading to the radiation of the pain in the head, neck, chest, shoulder, upper limbs and bowel and urinary disturbance in the lower part of the body. It is more common in females than in males.

Reasons: Cervical spondylosis predisposing factors may be trauma to the neck as is seen in road side accidents, boxing, karate, wrestling, car racing, cycling and during birth of the baby (like forceps delivery).

Various diseases like tuberculosis, rheumatoid arthritis may contribute to the development of this condition.

In today's time, sitting on the chair and working for long hours on computer, call-centre jobs, travelling for long hours in aeroplane or train in sitting posture and professionals working on table chair could add up for development of cervical spondylosis.

Sleeping in wrong posture may result in this problem.

Past neck surgery may also contribute to its development.

Presentation (Signs and Symptoms): Cervical spondylosis patients present with pain in the head (mainly occiput region), neck, arms and shoulder with or without movement.

At times, the referred pain is felt by the patients in the ears also.

Numbness, weakness and needle like pricking pain in the hands are often present.

Radiating pain and weakness in the arms and forearms is also present.

Bowel and urinary problems may be present in few cases.

On examination, the stiffness in the neck, shoulders and back muscles can be palpated.

Movement of the arms or neck is painful.

Ear examination is normal.

X-rays of the neck may show decreased disc space, osteophytes, osteoporosis and straightening of the cervical spine.

CT scan or MRI helps in clinching the diagnosis.

Treatment: Conservative management is the mainstay of treatment in cervical spondylosis.

Neck collar, physiotherapy (traction of the neck, short wave diathermy), neck massage with warm oil (mustard, olive, etc.), neck flexion and extension with side movement exercises, sleeping without pillow on firm bed without soft cushion, hot fomentation, pain relieving ointment and gels, analgesics helps in controlling the condition to a large extent.

Surgical management is the last resort which is usually done with laminectomy (removing the lamina portion of the involved vertebral bone) or anterior cervical discectomy with placement of bone graft in titanium cages.

Prevention: Professional activities, sitting on computers/laptop, travelling in trains or by air should not be done in one sitting posture but one should keep on moving in between and should engage in neck exercises while sitting also (like flexion, extension of neck and sideways movement of neck). This will prevent the development of cervical spondylosis.

Milk, calcium supplements and oestrogen hormone replacement therapy after menopause should be taken to prevent excessive loss of calcium from the body and occurrence of cervical spondylosis.

Yoga also helps in preventing its development by keeping the muscles and joints actively mobile. Hypertension, hypo or hyperthyroidism, diabetes should be treated well to prevent cervical spondylosis since these diseases may cause damage to the cervical spine.

Any sport activity should be accompanied with proper caution so that cervical spine is not damaged.

Vocal Cord Nodules (Teacher's or Screamer's Nodules)

Vocal cords are situated in larynx and helps in the production of voice.

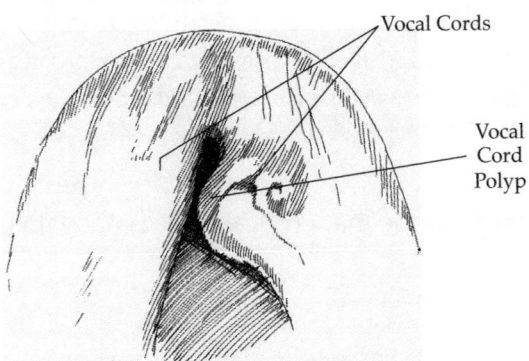

Vocal cords have vocalis muscle which is attached anteriorly to Adam's apple (Thyroid Cartilage) and posteriorly to Arytenoid cartilage.

Normally vocal cords lie in V shape position during breathing through which air keeps on moving in and out.

At the time of speech, vocal cords come together in midline and vibration of the vocal cords along with movement of the tongue and lips produced sound.

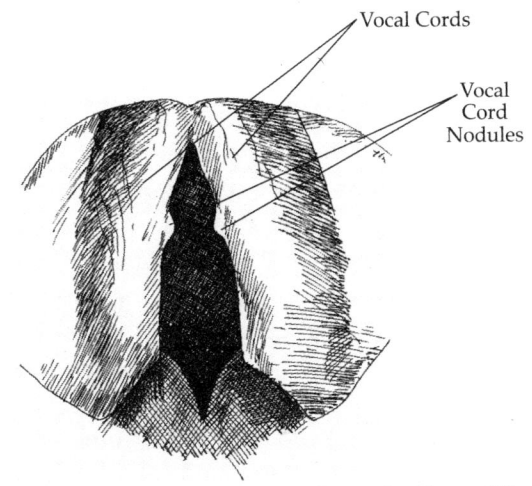

Fig. 3.3 Direct Laryngoscopy or Endoscopic View of Vocal Cord Polyp and Vocal Cord Nodules.

Vocal cord nodules are more common in females and these are found on both the vocal cords at the junction of anterior $1/3^{rd}$ and posterior $2/3^{rd}$ where maximum strain is present while speaking.

Reasons: Vocal abuse, speaking in louder tones for long periods as is seen commonly in singers, actors, teachers, politicians, etc. results in the development of vocal cord nodules.

Shouting, yelling, crying, screaming, etc. puts excessive strain over the vocal cords and leads to vocal cord nodules development.

Various diseases which affect vocal cords like tuberculosis, sarcoidosis, etc. can result in the development of vocal cord nodules.

Other contributing factors for the development of vocal cord nodules are allergy, smoking, chronic laryngitis, hypothyroidism (endocrine disorders) and gastro-oesophageal reflux disorders.

Presentation (Signs and Symptoms): Vocal cord nodules patients have symptoms which includes the hoarseness of voice, fatigueness of voice with sudden black out or complete loss of voice during prolonged speech.

Pain in the neck, head and ears are other associated symptoms.

Breathlessness, clearing of the throat often, husky voice may also be complaints of patients with this disorder.

On examination the throat may have pharyngitis, tonsillitis.

On indirect laryngoscopy or endoscopic examination with 45 degree or 70 degree endoscope, vocal cord nodules are seen at the junction on anterior $1/3^{rd}$ and posterior $2/3^{rd}$ of vocal cords.

These are usually pinkish-red in colour, small in size approximately pinhead to pea size, pedunculated (attached to the vocal cord by a small stalk).

Treatment: Conservative management with Broad spectrum antibiotics (like Cefpodoxime proxetil, Azithromycin, Sparfloxacin), Analgesics, Antihistamines, cough lozenges and Cough suppressants syrups may be required to treat pharyngitis, laryngitis or tonsillitis.

Voice rest, speech therapy and betadine gargles may also be helpful in treating the infection and managing the vocal cord nodules.

At times the nodules may resolve with the conservative management. If the conservative management fails, then surgical management with micro-laryngeal surgery (MLS) is performed. MLS is followed by speech therapy for 2 to 4 weeks.

Prevention: Vocal cord nodules can be prevented by stopping vocal abuse and speaking in softer voice. Changing the voice and mimicking in others voice should be avoided since it causes excessive stress on the vocal cords.

Smoking should be curtailed.

Hypothyroidism, tonsillitis and other chronic diseases should be treated in time.

Even after the surgery, voice abuse and yelling, shouting, screaming and crying should be avoided otherwise vocal cord nodules may recur.

Whiplash Injury to Neck

Whiplash injury to the neck is caused by the sudden extension of the neck as a result of accident and lead to severe pain in the head and neck region.

These injuries may cause damage to the tissues of the vertebral column in the neck which may get torn or stretched due to sudden jerky movement, forward and then backward.

Whiplash injury is mostly restricted to the spinal cord, involving the neck and chest region.

Reasons: Whiplash injury is most commonly caused by motor vehicles accidents from rear or back side in today's time.

In ancient time, falling from the back of horse while doing horse riding used to cause whiplash injury. Other causes of whiplash injury are sudden falling from chair backward, while playing football, doing aerobics, fall from height, dance with jerky head movements and assault.

Water sports activity, roller coaster rides, ice skating, river rafting, etc. may also cause whiplash injury in the modern world.

Presentation (Signs and Symptoms): The patients with whiplash injury presents with severe pain in the neck and head region.

The pain may also extend to the shoulders and arms with needle pricking sensation in the palms and fingers.

The ear pain and vertigo is often felt by the patients with whiplash injury.

The pain may be felt immediately after the injury or after a while; the earlier the pain felt, severe is the damage to the spine.

On examination, spasm is present in the muscles in the neck, shoulder and back region with pain on palpation.

Sideways neck movement are very painful.

Ear examination is otherwise normal.

Treatment: Conservative management with hot fomentation, analgesics with muscle relaxants, physiotherapy and local analgesic ointment and gels are the mainstay of the treatment.

Neck collar and bed rest should also be accompanied for faster recovery.

Prevention: Whiplash injuries can be prevented by driving properly so to prevent accidents on road. Immediate attention should be given to the injury and adequate bed rest and physiotherapy should be taken to prevent long term complications.

Children should be advised to take roller coaster rides, ice skating and other sport activities with care to prevent them from whiplash injury.

Artificial Dentures

Dentures are used to replace the old broken teeth.

These are commonly used in elderly individuals who are either edentulous or have lost few teeth.

With accidents becoming more common in today's time, artificial dentures are also fixed in younger individuals.

Reasons: Artificial dentures are put in after the natural loss of teeth with age and/or extraction of teeth due to caries.

After radiotherapy in the oral cavity for the cancer, the teeth may decay and artificial denture may be required to be put in after sometime.

Presentation (Signs and Symptoms): Artificial dentures may cause pain in the mouth, difficulty in mastication, ulceration in the mouth and radiating pain in the ears.

On examination of the oral cavity, denture removal may show congested gums and oral mucosa. Ulceration in the mouth may also be present.

Ear examination is more or less normal.

Treatment: Artificial dentures may be removed and better quality material denture may be replaced after few weeks.

Ulceration in the mouth may be treated with B-complex tablets.

Pain in the mouth and ear is treated with analgesics.

Analgesic gel may be applied in the mouth for local treatment.

Prevention: Soft food should be used initially for few weeks to months after the artificial dentures are applied in a patient.

Nutritious balanced diet should be taken to prevent ulceration in the mouth.

Good material artificial dentures should be used.

Pain in the Ear during an Aeroplane Flight

In today's modern era, air flights are common mode of transportation for local, national or international level.

With growing technology, availability of laptops and internet, people have easy accessibility of booking tickets online for travelling to different destinations.

The infrequent problem faced by the frequent traveller is ear ache which at times makes the passenger to abandon his trip by air.

At times, it makes the person scared of air travel also.

It is important that the passengers on board be explained the preventive measures for ear pain.

Reasons: The main reason for the ear pain during the flight is the air pressure difference between the external atmosphere and the middle ear (i.e. part medial to the ear drum).

Air pressure is maximum at the ground level and it decreases as we climb higher and vice versa. So in the aeroplane, the pressure is decreased during ascend and increased during descend to equalize the pressure.

During ascend, the air pressure outside to ear drum keeps on decreasing and middle ear pressure keeps on increasing which makes the ear drum to move inside.

Similarly during descent, the air pressure outer to ear drum keeps on increasing and makes the ear drum to move out resulting in pain.

Ear pressure balance is maintained by the eustachian tubes which connect the nose and throat to the ears.

Presentation (Signs and Symptoms): The symptoms are mainly pain in the ears, popping sensation, giddiness, vertigo, vomiting and headache seen in flyers.

Other associated symptoms of nasal congestion, running nose, sneezing, sore throat, fever and cough may be present in individuals with sinus or throat infection which may aggravate the ear pain.

Mainly the pain symptoms appear during descend since at that time, the pressure in the cabin is increased to equalize with the outside pressure and it is during descend that the ear drum tends to move outward with increased outside pressure than to the middle ear pressure.

During ascend when the outside pressure is less and the middle ear pressure is high then the ear drum moves inside which does not produce much pain or the pain generated is quite less.

On examination of the ear drum, the tympanic membrane may be congested, red, air bubble may be seen internal to the ear drum and some fluid collection may also be present medial to the ear drum. Other associated signs of congestion in the nose and throat may also be seen in affected individuals.

Treatment: In most of the individuals pain settles down after some time once the flight lands. In some of the individuals where heaviness, decreased hearing, blocked sensation in the ear and pain persists need for medication is present. Simple analgesics like paracetamol may be sufficient in mild cases. In some where associated nose and throat infection is also present, broad spectrum antibiotics like cefadroxil, cefuroxime axetil, cefixime and decongestants like xylometazoline nasal drops, loratadine, ebastine, levocetrizine, phenyephrine, etc. may be given. Mild steroidal nasal like flixonase sprays also have a good role in resolution of the nasal and ear symptoms.

Prevention: Ear pain in the aircraft while descend can be prevented by swallowing movements, yawning, drinking sips of water, cold drink at room temperature, juice, mildly doing valsalva manoeuvre, chewing gum.

The patients with nose and throat infection should consult an ENT specialist before boarding so to prevent the severe pain which may happen during flight.

Broad spectrum antibiotic (Cefpodoxime proxetil), Decongestant (phenylephrine), steroidal (Flixonase) nasal spray and pain killer (paracetamol) may be taken before the flight to prevent the severity of pain.

Use of Earphones

In Today's time, Earphones are commonly used by the teens and adults for the purpose of listening to songs on i-pods.

Bluetooth is the similar device used for talking wireless via mobile phones.

These earphones and bluetooth listening devices have reached in every nook and corner of the world. These do have beneficial purpose but there hazards can never be overlooked.

On one hand these give the liberty to hear songs on the move but on the other hand these cause irreversible damage to the vestibule-cochlear nerve (Nerve for hearing) due to high volume, longer duration and direct transmission of sound waves to the ear drum from the outer ear.

These newer advancements are a boon to humanity in terms of providing finer music and listening pleasure but there excessive usage should always be done with caution.

The new generation is mad about newer gadgets and consider it to be their pride and honour to flaunt it.

Though these devices are good to use off and on but should be curtailed on account of causing long term hearing loss.

Reasons: Use of earphones or earbuds is common with i-pods, i-phones, mobiles and other listening devices.

Hearing loud music above 85 decibels (dB) for more than 8 hours is harmful to the ears and can cause hearing loss.

Bluetooth earphones are used with mobiles for providing hands free, wireless listening and answering the calls.

Bluetooth earphones generate ultra high frequency (UHF) waves which are damaging to the internal ear and hearing nerve.

Presentation (Signs and Symptoms): The patients using earphones or Bluetooth earphones tend to have heaviness in the ears along with sensation of fullness in the ears.

They also have ear pain, headache, dizziness, hearing loss and vertigo.

Examination of the ears is unfruitful and do not show any positive findings.

Audiometry may show hearing loss mainly in higher frequencies (Acoustic Trauma).

Treatment: Stoppage of the usage of earphones should be done.

Antihistamines with mucolytic agents (Loratidine+Ambroxol, Cetrizine+Ambroxol) are the mainstay therapy for these patients.

Nose and throat infections should be treated as per requirement.

No surgical management is required in these cases.

Prevention: Minimal usage of earphones or Bluetooth earphones should be done. Any tinnitus, heaviness, decreased hearing, vertigo should be taken seriously and prompt management should be done.

Herpes Simplex of the Oral Cavity

Herpes simplex infection of the mouth is due to Herpes Simplex virus.

Herpes Simplex is of two types- HSV 1 and HSV 2.

Herpes simplex virus 1 (HSV 1) commonly affects the mouth, face, oral cavity, eyes and brain whereas Herpes simplex virus 2 (HSV 2) affect the anus and genital region and is sexually transmitted.

Herpes simplex of the oral cavity has symptoms including vesicular eruptions, weeping lesions on the lips, tongue, gums, buccal mucosa.

Reasons: Herpes simplex is a viral infection which spreads from one person to another via direct contact or through body fluids like saliva.

It remains latent in the nerves and has the tendency to recur. Recurrence occurs with decreased immunity, stress, fever, acute illness, exposure to sunlight and in persons on immuno-compromised drugs as is seen in malignancy, AIDS, etc.

Presentation (Signs and Symptoms): Herpes simplex infection comes prents with blisters and ulcers in the mouth, gums, lips, soft and hard palate and on buccal mucosa.

These start as small as maculo-papular lesions with red boundary which has clear fluid and these often break to release fluid and get converted to ulcers.

Patients with these ulcers tend to have severe pain in the throat, difficulty in swallowing their own saliva and pain radiating to the ears along with fever.

On examination of the oral cavity, round, ulcerated lesions are found in all the areas of the mouth starting from lips to the posterior part of the throat. These lesions may be present on face and in the eyes as well.

Often the lymph nodes are also enlarged and are tender on palpation.

Treatment: Herpes simplex lesions may be resolved on their own within 1-2 weeks.

Anti-viral therapy involving acyclovir, valaciclivir, famiclovir may be used for the treatment of the disease.

Supportive therapy with intravenous fluids, pain killers and nutritional supplements is often helpful.

Prevention: Herpes simplex can be prevented by avoiding the contact with the diseased individual.

Condoms are a good way to prevent sexually transmitted Herpes Simplex type 2. Stress should be dealt well by joining yoga and meditation classes.

Leucoplakia of the Oral Cavity

Leucoplakia is derived from the word "Leuko-" which means white and "-Plakia" which means patch.

Leucoplakia is the condition caused by tobacco chewing, and smoking which results in the development of whitish discolouration of the oral mucosa from pinkish red.

Leucoplakia may involve the female genital region also. This condition is a precursor to the development of oral cancer. Leucoplakia is usually seen in middle aged to older individuals.

Reasons: Leucoplakia of the oral cavity is usually caused by chewing tobacco, supari and smoking cigars, cigarettes, bidi, etc.

Nutritional deficiency (Vitamin A, B deficiency), alcohol, Candida fungal infection, Human Papilloma virus, Sharp teeth and AIDS may also be contributing factors for Leucoplakia.

The cause of Leucoplakia patches of the female genitalia is unknown.

Presentation (Signs and Symptoms): Leucoplakia of the oral cavity comes with difficulty in opening the mouth wider, mouth opening is limited and referred pain to the ear is also present.

Eating spicy, salty food is painful and is often restricted by the patient.

Bleeding from the gums and severe pain in the throat is present in severely affected individuals.

On examination of the throat, whitish patches are present on tongue, cheek, gums, soft palate, tonsils and posterior pharynx.

These white patches are well defined and are slightly elevated than the surrounding.

Ulceration of the mouth mucosa is also present with bleeding gums. Dental caries may also be present due to chronic tobacco chewing.

Treatment: Leucoplakia is treated by cessation of smoking, tobacco chewing and alcohol intake.

Nutritional supplements (B-Complex), Tablet Rebagen (Rebamipide), analgesic gels (mucopain gel), Lexanox gel, Tantum mouth wash and antacids (Rabeprazole) are given.

Steroidal injections and creams (Triamcinolone) are given in the mouth for the improvement in leucoplakia patches.

The treatment for Leucoplakia may be given for 6 months to 1 year.

Bland soft diet is also recommended in these patients. Sharpness of tooth and ill fitting dentures should be corrected.

Surgical excision of Leucoplakia patches may be done in the affected individuals who fail to respond to medical therapy.

Prevention: Intake of tobacco, cigaretees, bidi, supari, alcohol and cigars should be avoided at all cost.

After the diagnosis of Leucoplakia, complete cessation of intake of these things should be done to prevent the development of oral cancer.

Dental caries should be treated to prevent ulceration in the tongue and cheek. Misaligned teeth should be corrected.

GERD

Gastro-oesophageal reflux disease (GERD) is characterized by the reflux of the contents of the stomach in the oesophagus.

This causes heartburn, pain in the chest, sourness and pain at the back of the throat.

If the symptoms occur more than two times in a week then it is labeled as GERD.

With the advent of technology, rising pollution, contaminated food, water, air and tendency of levels individuals to do less walking and exercise, GERD is on the rise. It affects a good chunk of the general population more so in the higher class.

Reasons: GERD happens due to incomplete closure of the junction of stomach and food pipe leading to reflux of acid or acidic contents in the food pipe from stomach.

This may at times travel to the throat and gives rise to pain in the chest and throat.

GERD may also happen due to hiatus hernia where the stomach moves in the chest region due to defect or weakness in the diaphragm.

GERD may happen due to tumour in the gastrointestinal tract which secrete gastrin hormone leading to excessive acid secretion e.g. Zollinger-Ellison Syndrome.

Presentation (Signs and Symptoms): Gastro-oesophageal reflux disease comes with burning sensation in the chest, difficulty in swallowing, pain in the throat, acidic feeling in the food pipe, mouth and nose.

It may precipitate headache, change in voice, pain in the ears, feeling of giddiness and weakness.

Other symptoms attributed to recurrent ear, nose and throat infections may be due to GERD.

At times, the stomach contents or acid may be refluxed in the mouth or may partly come through nose. On examination, posterior throat wall may show congestion in GERD cases due to recurrent acidic reflux from the stomach. On endoscopy of the larynx, vocal cords and adjoining areas may be congested. Ear examination is usually normal.

Stomach endoscopy may show incompetency of the lower oesophageal valve, acid reflux.

Hiatus hernia may also be diagnosed on Upper Gastro-intestinal endoscopy.

Treatment: GERD is treated with medicines such as Rabeprazole (Rabifast), Omeprazole (Ocid), Ranitidine (Rantac).

Medicines which increase stomach motility such as Rabeprazole with Itopride (Rablet IT) helps in early stomach emptying thus decreasing the chances of acid reflux.

Digene gel, Mucaine gel helps in relieving the acidity by neutralizing the acid.

Hiatus hernia may be repaired surgically or otherwise sleeping with head and upper chest elevated with pillow or by raising upper part of bed elevation helps in reducing the symptoms.

Surgical excision of any tumour related with increased secretion of acid should be done.

Prevention: Acid reflux is the key to the GERD problem. It can be prevented by eating food in the night at least 3 hours before sleep, avoiding alcohol, tobacco chewing and smoking.

Milk intake acts as a good neutralizer for the acid and should be taken at night to prevent acid reflux.

Lying down or exercising immediately after taking heavy meal should be avoided.

Exercise, swimming, yoga, meditation and keeping stress at bay helps in reducing GERD.

Slightly elevated head and upper chest helps in preventing acid reflux so one can use pillows or elevate the head at end of the bed.

Too tight clothes should be avoided and loose clothes should be worn.

Weight loss in obese patients, sugar control in diabetics, intake of less oily meals and taking smaller meals helps in GERD.

Migraine

Migraine is the condition characterized by severe headache, nausea and vomiting preceded by an aura.

The headache persists for hours to days and is throbbing, pulsatile and unilateral.

Aura precedes headache for few hours to days and is the hallmark of most migraines.

Aura are the warning symptoms and these could be to increased sensitivity to light, sound or other sensory disturbances like needle like pricking sensation in the hands or palms, etc.

Migraine is more common in females than males.

Migraine has genetic preponderance and at times runs in the families.

Reasons: Migraine may be precipitated by certain food, beverages and alcohol.

Altering hormone levels especially in females is also considered to trigger migraine.

Migraine is said to develop due to decreased blood supply, neural hyperactivity in the brain.

Migraine may also develop due to stress, weakness, starvation, excessive hot or cold climate.

Presentation (Signs and Symptoms): Migraine comes with severe headache, usually on one side accompanied with nausea, vomiting and vertigo.

Aura usually precedes headache which could be photophobia (discomfort or pain in the eyes in the presence of light).

Visual aura is the most common which may manifest in patients with complaint of visualizing flashes of light, rainbow light, blurring of vision, tunnel vision.

Other sensory disturbances like phonophobia (uncomfortable with loud sounds), heaviness in ear, pain in the ear, tinnitus (voices in the ear), numbness or needle pricking sensation in the arms, hands or palms may also be seen.

Diarrhea, sweating, breathlessness, nasal blockage and excessive urination may also be present.

On examination, these patients have slight swelling of the face with visible pulsation in the arteries on the head on the affected side.

Neck stiffness and tenderness may be present. Ear and eye examination is within normal limits.

Treatment: Analgesics (Aspirin, Ibuprofen, Paracetamol), anti-emetics (Metoclopramide, Domperidone) are the mainstay of the treatment of Migraine.

Injectable steroids like dexamethasone may be used in some of the patients with acute symptoms. Caffeine is also advisable in these patients.

Surgical management with cauterization of the branches of the external carotid artery in the region of scalp may be done in confirmed cases.

Prevention: Migraine attacks may be prevented by maintaining a healthy lifestyle.

Special attention should be paid to manage stress by relaxing therapy, physiotherapy and regular exercise.

Preventive medicines like beta blockers or antidepressants may be used with caution in frequent migraine patients.

Food stuff, alcohol, smoking or other migraine precipitators should be avoided.

Chapter 4

Dos and Don'ts when you have an Earache

1. Impacted wax may cause earache and trying to clean it with the bud may push the wax inside resulting in increased pain, so one should not try to clean the ear by himself/herself.

2. Instilling warm or hot oil in the patient who has ear infection with intact ear drum may cause ear drum perforation, so one should avoid putting oil in the ear.

3. Swallowing movements help in reduction of the air pressure in the ear during the flight descend and is helpful in preventing the earache and decreasing the extent of earache. So one can sip water, juice, chewing gum, etc. to prevent the occurrence of ear pain.

4. Valsalva manoeuvre may increase the pain in the ear during descend, so it should not be done. Slight increase in the pressure in the middle ear

via valsalva may open the closed ear but should be done with caution.

5. Facial nerve stimulation treatment should be started immediately in cases of Bell's palsy (Idiopathic facial nerve palsy).

6. Facial nerve decompression treatment should be done at the earliest in cases of fracture of the Temporal Bone with facial nerve palsy or in chronic cases of ear discharge with facial nerve palsy.

7. Traumatic perforations should be handled conservatively and avoiding instillation of oil and ear drops helps in curing most of these cases.

8. During ear discharge, without consultation with an ENT specialist, instillation of antibiotic ear drops may lead to secondary infection with fungus in the ear.

9. Severe burning pain is followed by the eruption vesicles and blisters along the distribution of the branch of the facial nerve in Herpes zoster. It should not be misdiagnosed and should not be treated on the line of Staphylococcus Bullous Impetigo infection which may show similar presentation.

10. Trauma to the ear occurs in sports events like wrestling, cricket, boxing, judo, cycling, car race or martial arts. Most of these improve with proper

antibiotic coverage and pain killers. Don't do hot fomentation in these cases. Covering head with helmets prevent most of these injuries.

11. Road side accident injuries involving ears are treated with antiseptic dressings, antibiotics, analgesics, tetanus injections and surgery of the damaged ear, if required.

12. Acute tonsillitis or acute adenotonsillitis with ear pain is treated conservatively with broad spectrum antibiotics like cefpodoxime proxetil, azithromycin, cefuroxime axetil along with analgesics, anti allergics, anti pyretics, betadine gargles. In severe cases where swallowing of saliva is also difficult patients are admitted in the hospital and are given intravenous antibiotics, analgesics and intravenous fluids and supplements.

13. Don't take cold refrigerated products, spicy food, sauce, namkeens, etc. in patients with recurrent tonsils and adenoid infection.

14. Do regular brushing of the teeth to prevent earache due to dental caries.

15. Eating of candies, ice cream, chocolates, hot and cold liquids taken simultaneously spoil the hygiene of the teeth. This may result in dental caries with ear ache, so it should preferably be avoided.

16. Returning to the surface after scuba diving and sea floor walking should be slow so that pressure difference in the water and land does not cause headache or earache. Swallowing movements also helps in relieving pain and heaviness in the ears.
17. Apthous ulceration should be treated with B-Complex Syrup or tablets, Lexanox gel local application over the ulcers, Tantum mouth wash before meals and Betadine gargles with cold water after meals.
18. Control of Diabetes Mellitus is must in cases of Malignant Otitis Externa.
19. Don't try to treat Foreign Bodies in the ears at home. It may cause impaction of the foreign body.
20. Wearing artificial jewellery may aggravate the Dermatitis and pain in the ear. Avoid wearing nickel based artificial jewellery.
21. If a person is allergic to cosmetic cream, hair dyes, hair conditioner etc. then he should avoid the use of such substances.
22. Ulcerated, dry crusty or cystic lesion on the ear should not be scratched. This may be cancerous, especially in elderly individuals.
23. Quinsy or peritonsillar abscess should be treated with incision and drainage in hospital setting.

24. Hot fomentation and physiotherapy helps in relieving the pain in Temporo-mandibular syndrome.
25. Hard food or substances should be avoided and soft meals should be encouraged in Temporo-mandibular syndrome patients.
26. Neck collar, physiotherapy (traction of the neck, short wave diathermy), neck massage with warm oil (mustard, olive, etc.), neck flexion and extension with side movement exercises, sleeping without pillow on firm bed without soft cushion, hot fomentation, pain relieving ointment and gels, analgesics helps in cases with Cervical Spondylosis.
27. Professional activities, sitting on computers/laptop, travelling in trains or by air should not be done in one sitting posture but one should keep on moving in between and should engage in neck exercises while sitting also (like flexion, extension of neck and sideways movement of neck) to prevent development of Cervical Spondylosis.
28. Minimal usage of earphones as with I-Pod for listening music or bluetooth earphones as is seen with mobile phones for taking calls should not be done. Any tinnitus, heaviness, decreased hearing, vertigo should be taken seriously and prompt management should be done.

Chapter 5

Simple Tips to Take Care of Your Ears

- Never use ear buds at home to clean the ear, it will further push the wax inside and lead to impaction and pain in the ear.
- Use of warm oil (Olive oil, Almond oil or Mustard oil) may be used with caution under confirmed presence of wax in the ear. It helps in softening the wax in these patients.
- Hot fomentation of the infected ear (external or middle ear) further aggravates the problem and should be contraindicated.
- In children, when there is no obvious cause of crying, ear infection (otitis externa or otitis media) should always be ruled out by showing to the ENT consultant.
- Proper management of cough and cold i.e. acute adenotonsillitis, acute tonsillitis, acute sinusitis, acute pharyngitis, influenza helps in the prevention

of middle ear infection (acute otitis media) in most of the cases.

- Scuba diving, swimming, diving, sea floor walking, and air journey should be done with caution in patients suffering from cough and cold.
- Mothers should take care that breast or top feeding should be done with head in propped up position rather than in the lying down position to prevent milk going in the middle ear. They should also keep the child against their chest and make the child burp after each feed.
- Wearing helmets while boxing or wrestling prevents the development of cauliflower ear.
- Ear discharge may not be present in all cases of mastoiditis (Masked Mastoiditis) so even if the fever, hearing discomfort with pain behind the ear in the mastoid area is present then one should consult an ENT specialist.
- In advert use of antibiotic ear drops may lead to secondary infection with fungus, so instilling ear drops every now and then for itching etc. should be avoided.
- Fungal infection in the ear is seen in hot and humid climate. People involved in activities like swimming, sea walking, scuba diving, water sports, etc. are more prone to otomycosis.

- Usage of ear buds for cleaning the ear may traumatize the ear lining and may lead to secondary infection like otitis externa along with otomycosis.
- Facial nerve palsy in the discharging ear can be prevented by treating the ear disease at appropriate time. These cases should be operated so to prevent the spread of the infection to the facial nerve.
- Trauma to the ears may happen due to marital violence or household fights. Slapping on the face and ears is common by the husband on to the wife. Blunt trauma caused during such fights often results in ear perforation.
- Ear trauma may happen during fire in houses or factories.
- During road rage fights, people may beat each other or may bite the ear.
- Crawling of the insects like cockroaches, mosquitoes in the ears has also been associated with perforation of the ear drums.
- Adults while sleeping on the floor should cover their ears with a cloth or muffler or cap to protect themselves from the entry of mosquitoes or insects or cockroaches in the ears.
- Impaction of the foreign bodies like chalk, pencil lead, steel balls may happen if it is tried at home to remove them.

- If a person is allergic to cosmetic cream, hair dyes, hair conditioner etc. then he should avoid the use of such substances to prevent otitis externa.
- Strict maintenance of diabetes control is very important to prevent the occurrence of malignant otitis externa.
- The ear skin may produce allergic reaction following the contact with artificial jewellery (especially nickel containing ear rings or other jewellery).
- Tonsillectomy, adenoidectomy or functional endoscopic sinus surgery (in cases of Deviated Nasal Septum or Sinusitis) may be required to prevent spread of the infection from these sites to the ear.
- Ulcerated, dry crusty or cystic lesion on the ear should always be ruled out for the malignancy of the ear in elderly patients.
- Limited usage of mobile phones may be helpful in the prevention of Acoustic Neuroma. Tinnitus, deafness and headache symptoms should be dealt carefully in all the patients for early detection of the tumour.
- Trauma, frostbite, radiotherapy, psoriasis and actinic rays have also been instrumental in the development of cancer of the external auditory canal and middle ear.

- A small opening in front or on the ear i.e. preauricular sinus should always be looked in newborns and excised at an appropriate time.
- Cervical spondylosis presents with pain in the head, neck, arms and shoulder region and it should be ruled out in cases of ear pain.
- Ear pain in the aircraft while descend can be prevented by swallowing movements, yawning, drinking sips of water, cold drink at room temperature, juice, mildly doing valsalva manoeuvre, chewing gum.
- The patients with nose and throat infection should consult an ENT specialist before boarding so to prevent the severe pain which may happen during flight.
- Use of earphones or earbuds is common with i-pods, i-phones, mobiles and other listening devices.
- Hearing loud music above 85 decibels (dB) for more than 8 hours is harmful to the ears and can cause hearing loss.
- Bluetooth earphones are used with mobiles for providing hands free, wireless listening and answering the calls.

- Bluetooth earphones generate ultra high frequency (UHF) waves which are damaging to the internal ear and hearing nerve.
- Landline phones are a better option to prevent long term irreversible hearing loss which is seen with mobile phones and i-pods.